T0357170

I can think of no one who better understands people than Ian Cron. This book may be his most personal and his most pointed yet. Whether you have grappled with any kind of addiction, you love someone who does, or you just want to change something about your life, this is the book for you. Just picking up this book might be the half step you need in the right new direction.

Russell Moore, editor in chief, *Christianity Today*

Ian Cron's generous and hard-earned wisdom reveals that the Twelve Steps are not just for alcoholics and addicts; they are a path to a profound transformation of self for *everyone*. His guidance is practical and profound, offering a compassionate and joyful approach to recovery for all of us. Get *The Fix*, and you will get yourself back—with a newfound freedom to love and be loved by God and others.

Fr. Richard Rohr, O.F.M.

With *The Fix* comes a herald who pulls the curtain back on what we all sense in the deep: that we are people of insatiable longing, that our longing is often brutally and fathomlessly entangled with our pain, and that as a result, we are all addicts. But our author and guide does not leave us there. With the balm of humor that is required if we are to face the bracing reality of our lives as revealed on these pages and with a compelling vulnerability that never seeks its own notoriety, Ian Cron invites us all to come home. And home is where I want to be. Read this book, and begin to find your way there.

Curt Thompson, MD, psychiatrist and author
of *The Soul of Desire* and *The Deepest Place*

Ian Cron has written another book chock-full of spiritual insight, vulnerability, and humor. No matter who you are, this book will give you the tools to find hope, healing, and peace.

Bob Goff, author of the *New York Times* bestsellers *Love Does*, *Everybody Always*, *Dream Big*, and *Undistracted*

I feel compelled to tell you as a longtime endorser not just of Ian Cron's books but of Ian himself, *The Fix* should come with a warning label. This is not an inconsequential book. It will change your life immeasurably for the better—but only after first laying it bare. There's nowhere to hide here. Doesn't that sound, at least a little bit, like a relief?

Jen Hatmaker, *New York Times* bestselling author and host of the *For the Love* podcast

THE
FIX

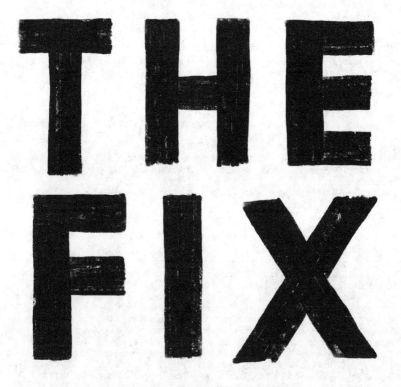

THE FIX

How the Twelve Steps Offer a Surprising Path
of Transformation for the Well-Adjusted, the
Down-and-Out, and Everyone In Between

IAN MORGAN CRON

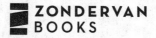

ZONDERVAN
BOOKS

ZONDERVAN BOOKS

The Fix
Copyright © 2025 by Ian Morgan Cron

Published in Grand Rapids, Michigan, by Zondervan. Zondervan is a registered trademark of The Zondervan Corporation, L.L.C., a wholly owned subsidiary of HarperCollins Christian Publishing, Inc.

Requests for information should be addressed to customercare@harpercollins.com.

Zondervan titles may be purchased in bulk for educational, business, fundraising, or sales promotional use. For information, please email SpecialMarkets@Zondervan.com.

Library of Congress Cataloging-in-Publication Data

Names: Cron, Ian Morgan, 1960- author.
Title: The fix : how the twelve steps offer a surprising path of transformation for the well-adjusted, the down-and-out, and everyone in between / Ian Morgan Cron.
Description: Grand Rapids, Michigan : Zondervan Books, [2025]
Identifiers: LCCN 2024036158 (print) | LCCN 2024036159 (ebook) | ISBN 9780310368540 (hardcover) | ISBN 9780310369288 (international trade paper edition) | ISBN 9780310368557 (ebook) | ISBN 9780310368564 (audio)
Subjects: LCSH: Twelve-step programs—Religious aspects—Christianity. | Spiritual direction—Christianity. | BISAC: SELF-HELP / Twelve-Step Programs | RELIGION / Christian Living / Personal Growth
Classification: LCC BV4596.T88 C76 2025 (print) | LCC BV4596.T88 (ebook) | DDC 248.8/629—dc23 /eng/20240904
LC record available at https://lccn.loc.gov/2024036158
LC ebook record available at https://lccn.loc.gov/2024036159

Cover design: Faceout Studio, Spencer Fuller
Cover illustrations: Shutterstock
Interior design: Kait Lamphere

Printed in the United States of America

24 25 26 27 28 LBC 5 4 3 2 1

To Aidan

CONTENTS

Chapter One

DESPERATE FOR A FIX

**What drives addiction is longing—
a longing not just of brain, belly,
or loins but finally of the heart.**
Cornelius Plantinga Jr., *Not the
Way It's Supposed to Be*

I was not born into a family of optimists. So one day, when I woke up to discover that my latest book—which my agent had said wouldn't sell, my mother had said wouldn't sell, and even I'd said probably wouldn't sell—was flying out the door, I was slack-jawed.

As my friend Derek and I were walking into a Barnes & Noble, he pointed to a front-of-store table with piles of my latest book on it. "Dude, you're blowing up," he said.

Yes, I was blowing up alright, but not in the way Derek thought.

Behind the mask of confidence, I felt like a fraud, as if I'd conned everyone else into believing I was worthy of my accomplishments when actually I was just a poser. I feared that people would soon discover I was an impostor and abandon me in disgust. And so, by 2020, I was secretly taking enough prescription medications every day to deaden my feelings of terror and self-doubt that you'd have thought my life's ambition was to become a mobile CVS pharmacy. Thankfully, a monthlong stint in rehab that same year prevented me from achieving that ill-considered goal.

"Prescription drugs? Rehab? How did this happen to you, Ian?" you might ask. "You're an Episcopal priest, a therapist, an author who writes books about spirituality, rewriting your life narrative, the mysterious workings of the personality and the human heart. You previously had decades of recovery from alcoholism. You have a nice home in a cool neighborhood in Nashville; you take vacations to Italy; you have two new cars in the garage. Dude, you even own goldendoodles. People who own goldendoodles don't take drugs and end up in treatment!"

Well, I did.

Repair Strategies

I'll soon provide you with all the unhappy details of my rack and ruin, doodles and all. How the reappearance of unruly ghosts from a difficult childhood, which I thought I'd put to rest, once again surfaced in my heart—like a jump scare from some mad uncle in the attic yelling, "Gotcha!"

But most important is what my relapse taught me: no matter how hard we try, we can't repair the enduring problem of the human condition—the pain of living in a world that's a colossal cock-up, a world that refuses to conform to our ideal of "how things should be," a world that repeatedly proves to us that our self-written prescriptions for soothing our emotional distress eventually cause us more problems than they solve.

Relapsing after decades of sobriety triggered a great deal of humiliation and shame. Now, years later, I still periodically wake up in the middle of the night and wonder, *WTF was I thinking?* All that said, it gave me one of the most important lessons of my life: my addiction wasn't the problem but only the symptom—I was in emotional, psychological, and spiritual pain and looking for "a fix," an external solution to an internal problem. This is a fool's errand, like going to the hardware store to buy bread. Our self-prescribed treatment plans for managing our own interior distress never, never, never work; they just keep us chasing the dragon, searching for the next "fix."

Which is why this book is about more than finding recovery from our addictions. It's a deeper exploration into the Big Ache that fuels addictions and other besetting self-defeating behaviors and how we can't fix it—at least not by ourselves. But this exploration will be teeming with hope because the solution to what ails us is always within reach and has been hidden in plain sight all along.

I begin with the assumption that you know you're broken. Why else would you buy a book titled *The Fix* if you weren't? Did you buy it for your partner? For your mentally maladjusted mother-in-law? No, you bought it for *you*—because there are days in your life that scare you, when you feel crazier than a rat in a dumpster fire. You secretly worry that if the authorities knew just how daft you were, they would pluck you out of the general population and place you in a secure location to protect the innocent. (Don't fret; you're not alone. I have so many disturbing voices in my head, my counselor has threatened to charge me for group therapy.)

Thankfully, most days you pass for harmless, along with the general populace of reasonably functional, garden-variety neurotics who can make fun of their kooky peculiarities and laugh them away. Yet if we're honest, we'll admit we can't banish the gnawing feeling that "something is rotten in the state of Denmark," as Marcellus warned in Shakespeare's

Hamlet.[1] We're uncomfortable in our own skin, in the world around us, troubled by a sensation of incompleteness—as if there really is a "hole in our soul," as countless spiritual masters have taught.

But we can't sit around on our bums all day fussing with our angst, so we repress these unsettling feelings or devise head-scratching strategies for exiling them to the land of shadows—that sunless realm beyond the fence-line of our awareness. Unfortunately, that murky sense of existential disease won't leave us alone. It follows us around like a feral cat wrapping its tail around our calves.

When the inner restlessness worsens, some of us begin to exhibit symptoms we, and sometimes others, can't ignore. We fall into misery-making patterns of crazy thinking, feeling, and behaving that baffle us and alienate us from ourselves and others. We become depressed, angry, anxious, lonely, and empty. Our relationships and work suffer.

So, what do we do? If you're like me and the rest of the huddled masses, you burn impressive numbers of calories trying to diagnose your own problem, as if naming it will endow you with magical powers to make it disappear. You go to therapy, attend self-growth retreats, practice yoga or mindfulness meditation, escape to a spa, take up Tai Chi, go on a diet (again), or read the latest self-help book that touts a miracle cure for what ails you.

Lord, have mercy, it's exhausting, right? I should know. I've tried every newfangled curative under the sun. (I even tried veganism once until it made me homicidal.)

So, what's our problem?

The Flaws in Our Best-Laid Plans

The Buddhists have a word that perfectly describes the human condition—*dukkha*. In Pali—an ancient language used in some Buddhist texts—this word translates to *suffering*, the source of which is a vague, underlying feeling of unease, inner lack, dissatisfaction, and inquietude. But I prefer how author and teacher Ethan Nichtern translates the word *dukkha* as the feeling of "not-at-home."[2]

Not since Adam and Eve were banished from Eden and the prodigal son flipped off his father have any of us really felt at home in the world. We are fractions yearning to become whole numbers. We have unnamable desires and unattended sorrows we don't know what to do with. We are filled with an inconsolable longing for what poet Anne Porter calls that "far-off and half-forgotten country . . . we half remember,"[3] and Christian apologist C. S. Lewis describes as a land we know exists, but "have never yet visited."[4] In short, you and I were made for paradise, but we feel like we're stuck in a Motel 6 on the border between heaven and earth.

This feeling of spiritual homelessness also shows up in the form of the inescapable pain that comes with living in a fallen world. We struggle with unresolved trauma, unfulfilled needs, grief, resentment, fractured relationships, self-contempt, a confidence deficit, insecurities that rob us of the lives we want to enjoy, and disappointment not only in ourselves but in those who we think should have loved us better but didn't.

"Life shouldn't be this way!" we cry.

No, it shouldn't. But here we are.

So, what are psychologically and emotionally limping

spiritual exiles like us to do when our self-repair strategies fail to solve our suffering?

We seek little "hits of pleasure" that distract us from facing our *dukkha* and numb the trauma from those million little emotional muggings we have experienced along life's way.

We spend hours in front of computer screens late at night watching porn while our family sleeps. We become technology addicts (sorry if you're reading this on your Kindle or iPad); control addicts; internet addicts; workaholics; relationship addicts; people-pleasing addicts; alcohol and drug addicts (I'll cop to both of those); drama addicts; video game junkies; sugar addicts; sex addicts; social media addicts; perfectionism addicts; status-seeking addicts; people who are addicted to the suffering of their past; sports junkies; plastic surgery addicts; tattoo addicts; Netflix addicts (curse you, *Seinfeld!*); shopping and spending addicts who have bumper stickers on the back of their cars that read, "I Brake for Garage Sales"; fantasy addicts; love addicts; rage addicts; "I need to be right" addicts; people who compulsively fix other people's problems (to avoid fixing their own); approval junkies; compulsive liars or exaggerators; caffeine addicts (cue grimace); nicotine addicts (I still miss it); worry addicts; compulsive helpers; exercise addicts; weight and dieting addicts; knowledge junkies; gambling addicts; news and politics addicts; money and security addicts; popularity addicts; self-improvement addicts; adventure-adrenaline addicts; productivity addicts; God and religion addicts (yeah, that's a thing); or food addicts—people like me who compulsively eat Fritos like they're mad at them or something.

Now listen, I understand if you skimmed over this onerously long catalog of troublesome behaviors. But sit with it for a moment and marvel with me at the bajillion self-medicating behaviors I left off it!

You know where I'm going, right? *We're all addicts.*

It's what humans do with their pain. No one's exempt—not even Mr. Rogers or the Dalai Lama. As psychiatrist Gerald May writes, "To be alive is to be addicted, and to be alive and addicted is to stand in need of grace."[5]

I used to consume heroic amounts of alcohol and prescription meds to relieve the pain associated with the aching feeling of "not-at-homeness" I felt in the world. I used substances to deaden unexamined pain from my childhood, to soothe the existential, free-floating anxiety that every human being must contend with. Beneath my chemical addictions lay my thirst for completion, for wholeness, for union with God, for peace with myself and others.

And what did I do?

I burned my life down to the ground.

Spiritual Workarounds

Chemical or process addictions (i.e., behavioral compulsions like viewing porn, gambling, spending, and countless others) are more than merely the deeply flawed means we use to avoid our half-cracked lives. They are also spiritual workarounds or shortcuts—self-designed strategies for making our lives more tolerable apart from reliance on the love, power, and grace of God. They consume our attention, drain our desire for the Divine, and attach it to idols, leaving us with less life energy to love other people, love ourselves, and love God.[6]

Which means addiction is another word for *sin*.

Now, before you have an apoplectic fit, let me offer a definition of that word that might sit better with you than the one you heard growing up from your creepy, snake-handling aunt. Richard Rohr writes, "Sins are fixations that prevent the energy of life, God's love, from flowing freely. . . . [They are] self-erected blockades that cut us off from God and hence from our own authentic potential."[7]

I may not entirely understand the doctrine of original sin, but I find it helpful to think of it as what I call the doctrine of original vulnerability. It helps us understand one of the reasons we have addictions in the first place. We're blasted into the furnace of life without adequate psychological defenses to fend off the unavoidable traumas, hurtful messages, and emotional injuries we all sustain in childhood. We then load these burdens into our little red Radio Flyer wagons and unconsciously pull them behind us into adulthood. Unfortunately, no one tells us how to heal these wounds. So, in adulthood, we end up developing chemical addictions, behavioral addictions, or recurrent self-defeating behaviors to cope with our dis-ease.

What makes it harder is that we live in a culture that normalizes and peddles addictive fixes. What better balm for the soul than the endless pursuit of material satisfaction? Advertisers and marketers have it down to a science. They know exactly how to hook us into believing their product or service will finally provide the fix for our inner turmoil. Years ago, I remember seeing an ad for a very expensive German sports car that proclaimed, "You can't buy happiness, but you can lease it." Or how about the T-shirt I once saw on an infant's onesie: "I'm the reason Mommy drinks wine"? (It's too bad there's no fix for stupid.)

And how many online marketing campaigns have you seen that appeal to our universal addiction to trying to control people, places, or things? Go ahead. Type "take back control of your life" into the search field on your computer's browser and see how many results pop up.

Don't worry, I'll be here when you get back.

Don't all these messages sound like a drug dealer's sales pitch: "The first taste is free, pal!"?

The reason we're powerless over our addictions is that—like alcoholism, drug addiction, or gambling—sin (addiction) is a disease. It's a deadly spiritual illness we inherited from our ancestors. Seriously, I wasn't consulted about the moral and spiritual shortcomings that were handed down to me. I've tried with everything in my power to defeat the potpourri of habitual sins, nutty self-limiting behaviors, and addictions that regularly torment me. Trust me, I'd empty my bank account if I could pay to get rid of even a handful of them. Alas, I can't. We can't control or overcome sin on our own unaided willpower any more than we can cure our own asthma. We need help.

Four mornings a week, I drag myself out of bed and go to a church basement where my boozy confederates and I sit in a circle on freezing-cold metal folding chairs to offer each other support as we recover from alcohol and drug addictions (and our many other fixations). Why? Because we have found a design for living that creates the natural soil in which we can grow in our relationship with God and so have the power to face the chronic sense of inner lack that landed us in that room in the first place.

I know firsthand what happens when we devise our own treatment plans to cure our spiritual homesickness on our own terms, without God's help. Bypassing God leads us to try other means of coping—the compulsive, self-defeating behaviors we use to anesthetize the Big Ache and make life more bearable *without God's involvement.* These strategies will eventually take us hostage. Take it from a guy who used to eat mood-altering substances like they were Tic Tacs—it's a really, really bad idea not to expose and dispose of your idols and adopt a new program of living to replace the one that's slowly (or not so slowly) cratering your life. God is the Great Physician, not us.

It can take ages before we realize just how much our addictions to things like food, drinking, work, trawling social media or doomscrolling the news on our smartphones, repeatedly returning to a hopelessly dysfunctional relationship, or any other compulsion is ravishing our emotional and spiritual life. As Gabor Maté says, "The attempt to escape from pain is what creates more pain."[8]

This is not what God had in mind for us.

The Bypass Tool of Denial

My later-in-life relapse came about because, in part, I forgot what life was like when I was in my active addiction years earlier. I began to think, *I've never been one of "those people." I've never curled up under a bridge asleep with a quart-sized plastic bottle of Smirnoff Vodka in my hands.* Oh dear, this is a well-worn script.

I had been in treatment for a week when I told my therapist, Jamie, "I've had some time to reflect on it, and I think my coming here was an overreaction. I'm sure my substance use isn't as big a problem as I thought it was. All I need is more self-discipline and a can-do spirit! I can go home and lick this thing on my own, right?"

Jamie smiled and said, "If I had a nickel for every addict who said that to me, I could buy Europe."

It took me a little while to warm up to Jamie.

This line of thinking is called *denial*, and everyone contends with this refusal to know what they know—that they have an addiction problem. Remember Faust? You know, the guy who made a deal with the devil? When he asked Mephistopheles, his visitor, who he was, he replied, "*I am the spirit who always denies.*"[9]

Addiction, like Mephistopheles, always denies that it's slinking around in your psyche laying waste to your life. It is the only disease that will daily tell you that you don't have a disease. In fact, your addiction gets a kick out of encouraging you to make New Year's resolutions or promises to yourself to give up whatever your fix of choice is because it knows you can't keep them—which, by the way, only makes your attachment to them stronger.

Unfortunately, denial often has a stronger grip on those with so-called "less obvious problems."

Let me explain. I remember attending my first Twelve-Step recovery meeting and hearing people introduce themselves by saying, "My name is so-and-so, and I'm a grateful recovering alcoholic."

Grateful? I thought. *Is this person still sozzled?*

But recovering chemical addicts like me have a reason to feel more grateful than people with secret, seemingly "less grave" addictions or crazy-making behavior patterns. My pharmaceutical misadventures eventually became glaringly apparent to family and friends, and I was eventually given the "you're becoming a socially indigestible sod" lecture and carted off to treatment, where I could find sobriety and recovery again. In rehab, I was afforded the luxury of time and support to uncover the "underlying causes and conditions" of the physical, emotional, and spiritual dis-ease that fed my addictions.

Sadly, people don't generally stage interventions for friends who are addicted to work, approval-seeking behavior, or the internet and send them somewhere where they can tend to their broken hearts and spirits and find freedom and joy. As a result, many people with less obvious but equally soul-killing addictions go to their graves without ever embarking on a healing journey.

I beg you—don't do that!

On Awakening

No one checks themselves into rehab because they're on a winning streak. At least I didn't. By the time I stumbled into treatment for my addiction to prescription drugs, I wanted nothing more to do with me. As my dear friend Mary says, "You know you've hit bottom when you break your own heart." Trust me, by the end of my last pharmaceutical jag, my heart was shattered.

When I first arrived at the treatment center nestled in the mountains of Utah, where I would spend the next thirty days working to recover the person I had lost, I'd hardly removed my coat before one of the staff people handed me a copy of *Alcoholics Anonymous* (a.k.a. *The Big Book*—the name I'll use from here on out) in which the Twelve Steps are laid out.

Perhaps you've heard of the Twelve Steps but don't really know what they are. The coauthor of the Twelve Steps was a hopeless alcoholic named Bill Wilson who found recovery as the result of a Damascus Road–like spiritual experience in a hospital room where he was dying from alcoholism. From that day forward, Bill never drank again.

The Twelve Steps derived from the teachings of a Christian organization called the Oxford Group, but Wilson rewrote them in such a way that people, regardless of their religious background or spiritual orientation, could benefit from them. What Bill Wilson came to understand was that the addict's problem was principally spiritual, not psychological or moral, and therefore required a spiritual solution. Thus, the purpose of the Twelve Steps was to enable alcoholics (or anyone else who wanted fixing and a better life) to have a spiritual awakening. Here's an amended version of the Twelve Steps. I've left the word *alcohol* out of the first Step so you can insert your chemical or behavioral "fixes of choice."

1. We admitted we were powerless over _____
   —that our lives had become unmanageable.
2. Came to believe that a Power greater than ourselves could restore us to sanity.

3. Made a decision to turn our will and our lives over to the care of God as we understood Him.

4. Made a searching and fearless moral inventory of ourselves.

5. Admitted to God, to ourselves, and to another human being the exact nature of our wrongs.

6. Were entirely ready to have God remove all these defects of character.

7. Humbly asked Him to remove our shortcomings.

8. Made a list of all persons we had harmed, and became willing to make amends to them all.

9. Made direct amends to such people wherever possible, except when to do so would injure them or others.

10. Continued to take personal inventory and when we were wrong promptly admitted it.

11. Sought through prayer and meditation to improve our conscious contact with God as we understood Him, praying only for knowledge of His will for us and the power to carry that out.

12. Having had a spiritual awakening as the result of these Steps, we tried to carry this message to alcoholics [our fellow sufferers], and to practice these principles in all our affairs.

Don't worry if your first read of the Twelve Steps makes you think, *This is the fix? It seems too simple.* Well, thank Almighty God for that! The Twelve Steps were written in such a way that anyone, regardless of their social or educational background, could understand and work them.

People in recovery often say, "It's a simple program for complicated people." This Enneagram Four wouldn't be sober today if this weren't the case.

More importantly, the Twelve Steps aren't snake oil. Lord forbid they become another wellness hack that those preternaturally attractive people wearing wide-brimmed hats blather about on TikTok. The Twelve Steps is a proven program that has literally saved millions of lives since these Steps were first published in 1939. All to say, there's oodles of evidence that they can deliver on their promise to profoundly transform the human heart.

According to Bill Wilson, if you committedly "work the Steps," you will eventually have a vital spiritual experience that will give you an entirely new and radically beautiful orientation toward life. When practiced as a way of life, they can expel your addictions and recurrent self-defeating behaviors and give you a "new pair of glasses" through which you will see yourself, others, and the world in a startlingly fresh way. The Twelve Steps will displace the broken old ideas that were once the guiding force of your life and replace them with a whole "new set of conceptions and motives."[10] This renewed relationship with God or a "Power greater than ourselves" will reconfigure your personality (your all too predictable and habitual patterns of thinking, feeling, acting, and interpreting your experience of the world) and render your addictions unnecessary.

The Steps don't just help a person abstain from a substance or habitual self-limiting behavior, *though that's obviously the first order of business*. More importantly, they address the underlying emotional, spiritual, and psychological issues that caused the addiction in the first place. The aim of the Twelve Steps is to draw us as close to God, ourselves, and others in this lifetime as possible. They teach us how to live joyfully in a riven world where we will never feel quite at home. They work.

Furthermore, the Steps are not abstract concepts, but straightforward and practical. They are not liberal, conservative, Protestant, Orthodox, Catholic, Muslim, New Age, or Zoroastrian. You can be a Christian, a Jew, a Zen Buddhist, or an agnostic flat-earther and benefit enormously from working the Twelve Steps.

I'm a "Jesus guy," but some aspects of my tradition make my teeth hurt. Christianity is often long on "the what" but short on "the how." For instance, contemporary Christianity is often primarily a *belief-based* religion in which salvation is found merely by offering assent to a set of theological propositions.

The genius of the Twelve Steps is that it's predominantly a *practice-based* program that brings about the profound psychological and spiritual shift that mere intellectual belief in God cannot. Moreover, the Twelve Steps are completely consistent with the gospel. They put wheels on the teachings of Jesus. They transform faith from a belief system into a lifestyle.

For me, the Twelve Steps have made me a better follower of Jesus. They have complemented and illuminated my understanding of the gospel; I know scores of Christians in recovery who would say the same thing. Given how helpful they are for the Christian, I'm amazed at how long the church has overlooked them as a design for living.

I have a pal named Gene (not his real name) who was fired from his role as senior pastor of a large, theologically conservative, nondenominational congregation for showing up drunk to church one Sunday. (I would have paid a hundred bucks for a front seat to that show.) He was only a minute or two into his slurred sermon when the elders realized he was completely potted and escorted him out of the sanctuary. There were no altar calls that week. Sadly, rather than help Gene find help, his church showed him the door.

One night after a meeting, he said to me, "Isn't it ironic that I have found more grace, forgiveness, acceptance, and healing in the basement of churches where Twelve-Step recovery groups meet than I ever did upstairs in the sanctuary where so-called 'normies' gather to worship? I wish they knew what they're missing!"

Now, here's the good news. Bill Wilson said that the Twelve Steps offered a spiritual solution for not only the alcoholics and addicts meeting downstairs in the church basement but also for everyone upstairs in the sanctuary and beyond who is searching for "home"—a solution to the Big Ache—which is all of us. I have seen the Twelve Steps unscrew countless people's screwed-up lives. And, yes, you can be one of them.

The Promise of Recovery

A Twelve-Step program is not a quick fix; it's a way of life. You don't work through the Steps once; you draw on their wisdom every day. This miraculous program isn't only for alcoholics, drug addicts, or for people trapped in recurring cycles of self-damaging behaviors; it's also for *anyone* who is "sick and tired of being sick and tired"—those who want to stop doing things to make themselves feel better that eventually do more harm than good, who desperately want to learn how to live healthily in a world that doesn't feel quite right, who want to heal from their old wounds rather than resort to hidden or obvious addictions to try to numb or distract themselves. It's for folks who want to be free to love God, themselves, and others.

In this book, I'm going to tell you about a genuine, time-tested, evidence-based, Spirit-inspired "fix." It's not the failed quick fixes you currently subscribe to. In applying the Twelve Steps to your life, I'll show you the fix that can break you out of the prison of your addictions, warped thinking, and quackish behaviors, one that will finally help you get your life together the way you were meant to live it. In other words, I wrote this book to help you find recovery.

Recovery is a word you're going to see pop up in this book repeatedly, so let me tell you what it means for me. Recovery has meant infinitely more than learning to give up mood-altering substances and behaviors. That's just the beginning! If the terms *addiction* and *sin* are synonymous, then for me, the word *recovery* is interchangeable with the word *salvation*.

People often get all worked up when I tell them I believe Christianity is an enlightenment religion. But isn't the point of our faith journey to become filled with the light of Christ? For me, as a Christian, the goal of recovery is enlightenment, to enjoy the marvelous adventure of a divinely directed life, to have a daily reprieve from my addictions, and to become truly useful to God and of service to my fellows. I think my friends who come at the Twelve Steps from other spiritual points of view would agree with me.

In my experience, recovery is all about what you do with your pain and emptiness. Will you numb it and slowly (or quickly) shipwreck your life? Or will you learn to walk with God in the often-painful tension of it all? Recovery is about discovering or rediscovering God in a way that will interrupt the circuit on your self-destructive behaviors and addictive strategies for making your life more tolerable. It is a new state of consciousness.

Unless you vacation in Sedona or you're into drum circles and crystals, you may not thrill to the idea of realizing a "new state of consciousness." But what if I told you it's the only way to satisfy the deepest longings of your soul for the fix it needs but can't get for itself? In the next chapter, we'll look at the ways chemical or process addictions offer a false fix for these deepest longings. Addiction feeds you the lie that it can fix those longings by temporarily deadening the pain or drawing your attention away from it.

Now, to be clear, this is not a self-help book (if your "self" could have helped your "self," wouldn't your "self" have done it by now?). I suspect you've repeatedly tried to overcome your addictions and negative habitual behaviors on your own and have discovered it didn't work. There's a reason for that. We don't heal ourselves. We heal each other.

Interestingly, the pronoun *I* appears nowhere in the Twelve Steps. Everything is written in the first-person plural. That's because recovery is a "we," not "me," proposition. You can't overcome your addictions and live this new way of life without help. This highlights how important it is for anyone embarking on a journey of recovery to find a Twelve-Step community of people who will walk alongside them on the path toward a life of healing and sobriety.

For some people, finding this community will be easy.

There are hundreds of Twelve-Step fellowships that address different addictions, compulsions, mental health challenges, or self-defeating behaviors. You can hop on the internet and look up a program and meeting times for the Twelve-Step group that focuses on your particular addiction or self-medicating behavior.

Once you're connected to a Twelve-Step recovery community, try to find a sponsor as quickly as you can. A sponsor is a person who has been around the program for a while who can guide you through the Steps and help you navigate early recovery. Throughout this book, you'll hear me talk a lot about my sponsor, Steve, and how much I've come to rely on his wisdom over the years. May you all find your own "Sponsor Steve"!

Okay, now don't go all wibbly-wobbly if you're not ready to check out a local Twelve-Step group yet. Start small. Ask one or two friends if they'll read this book (and workbook!) and explore the Twelve Steps together with you. You can do that, right?

Now, one last thing. My somewhat recent fall off the wagon might make you ask, "Why should I listen to this backslid delinquent?" Or, "How could a reputable publisher give this guy a contract to write a book on *any* topic, much less one that's about Twelve-Step spirituality and putting your life back together?" Heck, I've asked these questions too.

I'm not an addiction counselor. I'm not an expert in the neuroscience of addiction. I'm not a clinical psychologist who specializes in treating people with substance use disorders. But my relapse and the solution I found for it are still fresh and vivid in my mind. My friend Becca reassured me,

"Your relapse didn't erase everything you previously learned over thirty years as a priest and therapist or a person in recovery. Maybe you have more wisdom to offer now than ever."

I'm in no position to evaluate that statement, but I can say that what I've gleaned from living a life organized around the Twelve Steps is worth more to me now than ever. Otherwise, I wouldn't have asked you to join me on this adventure.

All to say, if you don't mind walking alongside a gimpy guide who can accompany you on the road to recovery, then I'm your guy.

"There is a solution," Bill Wilson famously wrote of this spiritual awakening near the beginning of *The Big Book*.[11] This solution is yours—and mine—for the taking, my new friend. Read on, and let's find out how.

Chapter Two

DRINKING FROM THE WRONG WELL

Every addiction starts with pain and ends with pain.
Eckhart Tolle, *The Power of Now*

I hail from a long line of hard-drinking, barroom-brawling Irish Catholics who believed that Budweiser, Marlboro Reds, and making regular visits to the ER for sutures equated to "living your best life."

This is how I describe my family to people who ask me about my upbringing, and I always want to hear a drummer follow it up with a rim shot to punctuate the joke. But my facetious answer is a psychological defense, a way of rolling the turd in glitter. It's a strategy to avoid having to admit that my family history is more harrowing than hilarious.

My grandfather was probably an alcoholic who, my father bragged, "mixed the meanest martini in New Rochelle, New York." This always struck me as a strange point of pride. My father himself was a chronic alcoholic and Valium addict, who died at sixty-two from way too many years of hard living. How he survived for so long after suffering alcohol-related liver disease, multiple esophageal ruptures, regular falls down staircases on Christmas and Easter mornings, and a catalog of other besotted catastrophes boggles the mind. And if that weren't enough, I have more than a smattering of other close relatives who died from drinking, and today I have several family members who are either in recovery or who I pray will be soon.

All to say, addictions don't run in my family—they gallop through it.

Alcoholism and drug addiction—what the *Diagnostic and*

Statistical Manual of Mental Disorders (*DSM-5-TR*) now politely calls "substance use disorder"—is a fiendish and widely misunderstood condition. Contrary to what many believe, addiction is neither a moral failure nor a condition that only afflicts the weak-willed. It is a disease of the body, mind, and spirit. Trust me, no one gets up in the morning, looks in the mirror, and says, "Today I'm purposely going to drink, overeat, or watch so much porn that I eventually shred my life into little bits of colored paper and shoot them out of a confetti cannon." I should know. That's precisely what I came close to doing before I first went into recovery from alcoholism on February 14, 1987.

In Twelve-Step recovery meetings, one often hears alcoholics and addicts say that for as far back as they can remember, they felt different from other people, as if they were born missing something important and unnameable in their essential makeup.

Lord knows, I did. I was a pint-sized, sensitive, artistic, and spiritual-minded kid who loved songwriting, poetry, journaling, the mystery of the Catholic Mass, thinking about the ultimate questions of life while wandering alone in the woods, and reading books that far surpassed my grade level (what ten-year-old reads Tolstoy's *Anna Karenina*?). I was a sweet, albeit precocious, child who felt separate from the herd and anxious, like I was wearing my skin inside out. To make matters worse, my crazy home life only aggravated my sense of apartness.

My Self-Medicating Fix

How did I deal with this feeling of not being at home in the world? Given how big of a deal alcohol was in our house, it made sense that I became fascinated by it from a young age. Beginning around age eight, I would sneak gulps from the decanter of Dewars Scotch my father kept on a side table in our living room (making sure no one was around), because it made me feel the way a kitten does when you stroke its tummy.

The first time I actually got drunk, though, was on a snow day in the eighth grade with a group of guys at my friend Grant's house. My friends drank only enough to get tipsy. Not me. I threw back so many orange Tangs-with-vodka cocktails that I ended up being raced to the hospital for alcohol poisoning. Though I have only a vague memory of this episode, I do remember feeling that the more I drank, the more my unrelenting self-consciousness and sense of disconnection disappeared. This was a harbinger of things to come.

My behavior did not sit well with my no-nonsense mother, who grounded me for a year. This wasn't an idle threat. She insisted I drop my "brainless" friends, and for the next twelve months, she made me come home immediately after school every day, where I did my homework and listened to my older brother's records. But she needn't have worried that I would be a repeat offender, at least not yet. My experience at Grant's house scared me so much that I vowed never to drink again, a promise I kept until tenth grade. But the pledge did nothing to address the underlying reason that made drinking attractive. That said, I found other forms of mood-altering entertainment to replace Todkas (the name I gave my drink of choice). I began smoking weed and unfiltered Camels, sexually acting out, and doing anything else that might relieve me of the burden of being me.

My drinking accelerated in high school, and I became the kind of guy who would steal your wallet and then help you look for it. My reputation for partying earned me the dubious nickname "Johnny Walker Red." I felt proud of that moniker when I was sixteen. But in hindsight, I wish I had earned a more innocent sobriquet, like Huck or Chip. Though I drank heavily in my mid-teen years, I wasn't the kind of drinker who got hammered every time I drank. Even so, I couldn't predict what would happen once I started. There were nights when I would go out and drink a few beers and go home, and other times when I'd go to a bar in Connecticut and wake up the next morning in a strip mall parking lot in Foster, Rhode Island.

Over time, my drinking continued to spiral downward. Though I was underage, I would go out alone nearly every night to a workingman's bar called the Lucky Charm where I would drink, eat dinner, and, strangely enough, do my homework. The drinking age was eighteen in those days, but Sal the owner wasn't a stickler. He'd have served me rubbing alcohol on the rocks with a twist if I had flashed him my library card and a ten-dollar bill.

My Religious Fix

At the end of my junior year, a girl I liked took me to a Young Life meeting, a nondenominational Christian organization for high school kids. I soon became a Christian, which greatly complicated my life.

I became two people, with two wildly different groups of friends and social calendars. When I wasn't hanging out at the Lucky Charm, I was at a Bible study or a Young Life club meeting where kids held hands and tearily sang Simon and

Garfunkel's "The Sound of Silence." Like the lives of lots of budding alcoholics, my life was becoming increasingly secretive, contradictory, and compartmentalized.

When I graduated from high school, I went to Bowdoin, a small New England liberal arts college in Maine, where I immediately joined a notoriously bacchanalian fraternity and the campus Christian fellowship in the same week. My sister was a successful cover girl model for the exclusive Eileen Ford Agency in New York in those days. Flush with money and VIP status, she would fly me from Maine to Manhattan where we'd spend weekends clubbing at the Limelight and CBGB. It became increasingly difficult to juggle faith and foolery, but it never occurred to me that I could live another way if I chose to.

For the next four years, I drank loads of beer from bong funnels on Saturday nights, danced alongside Truman Capote at Studio 54, and then attended prayer meetings on Sunday nights. I wore so many faces that I had no idea which was the real me.

When I graduated from college, I returned to my hometown, where I tried to settle down and grow up a little. I became a volunteer for the local Young Life club while maintaining a close friendship with three fellow Irish Catholic pals from high school who also came from unstable homes and were well on their way to becoming alcoholics. I have no idea where I got the money in my early twenties, but the four of us went out bar crawling every night. We never won "citizen of the year" awards, but we earned high marks for consistency.

In 1987, I married my college sweetheart, Anne, which upended my secretive drinking routine. As a Young Life staff member, I became a pro at masking my struggles with drinking. I was a deft chameleon who could project different personas as needed and make it work, but inside I knew that my life had become an unsustainable charade. I wanted to be a deeply spiritual person and a supportive husband, but I still didn't know how to address the deep pain within. So I continued to numb out through drinking. I began hiding alcohol around the house, going to bars alone in other towns to avoid being seen by the parents of my Young Life kids, and sneaking drinks before I went out with friends so I could get a head start and not look like I was out of control in front of them. When I wasn't drinking, I was thinking about drinking.

My inner world soon became increasingly dark and chaotic. My drinking and unaddressed childhood trauma were catching up to me. I fell into a deep depression, began to have panic attacks, and didn't want to leave the house.

On my doctor's recommendation, I went to see a therapist named Dan, who, unbeknownst to me, was a recovering alcoholic. We had been meeting for a brief time when Dan told me he wouldn't see me again until I sought help for my drinking. But, as Anne Lamott says "Trying to reason with an addict was like trying to blow out a lightbulb."[1] I angrily told Dan I wasn't an alcoholic and stormed out of his office.

I finally hit rock bottom a few weeks later on New Year's Eve when my wife, Anne, and I went to a party at my sister's apartment in Manhattan. This has become known as the Night of the Living Dead. I will not go into all the sordid details of what happened that night, but I'm told it involved my drinking a magnum of champagne, Homeric quantities of a Scandinavian drink called aquavit, nearly getting into a fistfight at a swanky restaurant called The Odeon, throwing up and blacking out in the back of a limousine, and waking up the following morning in Connecticut with a supernaturally cruel hangover.

Anne reached the end of her tether and insisted I go back to see Dan. By this point, I was exhausted from being chased around the paddock by the Four Horsemen of addiction—Terror, Bewilderment, Frustration, and Despair—to do whatever it took to get well. God bless him, Dan agreed to see me again and took me to my first Twelve-Step recovery meeting.

My Sobriety Fix

Thankfully, my obsession with drinking was immediately lifted, as so often happens to folks when they enter the rooms of recovery. The problem is I never really "got" the program. Sure, I learned about the Steps, but I never wholeheartedly threw myself into working them. I ventured in and out of the rooms. I dabbled in recovery.

That said, the years that followed were wonderful. Anne and I had three beautiful kids; I received a master's degree in counseling psychology and a Master of Divinity degree. I founded a church, became an Episcopal priest and spiritual director, moved to Nashville, wrote a few books, and became a songwriter, among other things.

But an addiction never completely goes away. I remember once attending a Twelve-Step meeting and hearing a speaker say that while we were sitting there, "our addiction was in the parking lot doing pushups and getting stronger." It's always in the shadows drinking protein shakes and waiting for an opportunity to wreak havoc, even after lying dormant for decades. You have to stay vigilant. I didn't. I felt I had my addiction licked.

What I failed to recognize is that my addiction didn't stem from my problem with alcohol or drugs. No, it came from my problem with *living*. I was an explosive waiting to go off. It had a long fuse, because for many years I was able to get away with the pretense that I no longer had those problems with living— things were going better than ever, it seemed. But eventually my hidden pain, fear, and resentment detonated. Just when I thought I was doing pretty well with living, I blew my life up.

My Adderall Fix

It all began with a visit to my doctor's office, where I had gone for my annual physical. While speaking with the doctor, I spied an amber-colored plastic prescription bottle on his desk with the words *amphetamine salts* printed on the label. For reasons I'm only beginning to understand, the little addict inside my head awoke from decades of hibernation and said to himself, *Wait, amphetamine salts? Doctors actually dole those out to people? How interesting . . .*

And so, without any premeditation, I went fishing. "Dr. Williams, what do you prescribe amphetamine salts for?" I recall, hissing like Gollum. (Okay, I probably didn't sound like Gollum, but I remember it that way.)

"It's the generic name for Adderall," Dr. Williams said, not bothering to look up from the script he was writing for me on his pad.

Obviously, as a therapist I knew about Adderall, a powerful stimulant prescribed to people with ADHD, but I also knew that in some shady circles, Adderall was code for "speed."

Lots of people who abuse Adderall without a prescription think it's merely a performance-enhancing drug that makes it possible to read and write a paper on James Joyce's *Ulysses* in under two hours. But Adderall is far from a harmless drug, particularly for people like me who have a history of addiction. Most folks don't know it, but Adderall appears alongside drugs like oxycodone, morphine, fentanyl, and codeine on the FDA's schedule II list of controlled substances because of its "high potential for abuse which may lead to severe psychological or physical dependence."[2] As a therapist, I knew enough about ADHD that I could recite aloud the criteria one needs to meet to be diagnosed with the condition. Now fully committed to "jumping on the A-train," I proceeded to try to fool Dr. Williams into believing I suffered from ADHD, which, by the way, I definitely do not. I justified this by thinking, *Maybe it will help me get more done.*

To my amazement, I pulled the wool over the kind and unsuspecting Dr. Williams's eyes. Thirty minutes later, I walked out of his office with a prescription for Adderall, along with another for Xanax and later Klonopin, two potent and highly addictive sedatives normally prescribed for anxiety, but meds I eventually used to cool my engines when I dosed too much Adderall.

It didn't take long before I was daily taking far more Adderall, Xanax, and Klonopin than what I had been prescribed—I mean, a lot more. I began to carry one pocket full of Adderall and one pocket full of Xanax or Klonopin and would titrate them all day. When I walked down the street, I sounded like a pair of maracas.

I won't make you suffer through the details of all the regrettable things that happened as a result of my doing pharmaceutical speedballs—how I once lost twenty-five pounds in thirty days; the damaging effect it had on my relationships with family members, friends, and work colleagues; and how I began lying to doctors to get more prescriptions ("the dog ate my toiletry kit"). It's still hard for me to believe I did those things.

And here's the crazy thing: did any of those frightening, adverse consequences strike me with sufficient force that I was ready to admit I was powerless and that my life was unmanageable—Step One of the Twelve Steps? Heck, no! "I can give it up anytime I want to," I told myself, "as long as it's next Tuesday." Sadly, I needed to go out and "conduct a little more research" before I finally pulled my chute and checked into treatment.

The Ultimate False Fix

Millennia ago, the Hebrew prophet Jeremiah spoke truth to the power of addiction: "My people have committed two sins: They have forsaken me, the spring of living water, and have dug their own cisterns, broken cisterns that cannot hold water" (Jeremiah 2:13).

That's right, I drank from the wrong well.

To be honest, drugs initially worked like a charm. They often do at first. Mood-altering chemicals anesthetized the ever-present feeling of homelessness. Highly addictive sedatives like Xanax and Klonopin calmed my anxiety and the sense that I didn't belong anywhere or to anybody. Amphetamines made me feel euphoric and unstoppable when I was feeling sad and lost.

But the universe has rules, people, and you can only bend them so far before they eventually snap back and punch you in the face. As I said in the previous chapter, I eventually ended up at an amazing treatment center in the mountains of Utah. There I learned something new: none of us has only one addiction; we are all boiling cauldrons of addictions.

I discovered I wasn't addicted just to substances; I was also addicted to controlling people, places, and things. I was hooked on seeking credentials and titles, on needing to be the smartest guy in the room, on notoriety, and on winning the approval of others, *to name only a few*. Seriously, I can't get out of bed and walk to the bathroom in the morning without stubbing my toe on one of my many addictions. I realized I had a lot of work to do, and that achieving sobriety in every area of my life would be a lifelong challenge. As author Anne Lamott puts it, "Getting all of one's addictions under control is a little like putting an octopus to bed."[3]

Today addictions are epidemic. The statistics on chemical and process addictions are enough to make you want to light your hair on fire and run around the neighborhood begging your neighbors to cut it out. Research predicts that the spike in excessive drinking during the COVID-19 pandemic may trigger consequences by the year 2040 of eight thousand more deaths from alcohol-related liver disease, nearly twenty thousand more cases of liver failure, and one thousand more cases of liver cancer.[4] As Brené Brown noted nearly fifteen years ago in her research about vulnerability, "We are the . . . most addicted and medicated adult cohort in US history."[5]

Okay, what precisely is an addiction and how does it start (oh, and end . . .)?

How Addiction Works

Many people I know cannot accept the idea that everyone is on the addiction continuum, that even our smallish hidden compulsions are obstacles to intimacy with God and the experience of a full life. But to believe this flies in the face of historic Christian teaching. Even the fourth-century Christian desert mothers and fathers spoke about the perils and universality of addiction, only they called them *attachments*. According to these spiritual teachers of the early church, an attachment is a physical, emotional, or psychological dependence on "some real or illusory object" that eventually robs a person of their freedom. We can know we are in the grip of an attachment when we use it "in excess of our needs, for purposes other than that for which they were intended, as ends rather than as means to a legitimate end."[6]

One of my favorite parables about addiction—an old story about a skylark, a bird known for its singing while in flight—nails the often sneaky and insidious process of getting hooked.

Once upon a time, there was a skylark that was particularly fond of worms and would give anything to get them. One day, as she was singing in the sun, she looked down and noticed an old man in a tiny coach who was shouting, "Who will buy? Who will buy? I am selling in all weathers fine and fat and juicy worms in exchange for skylarks' feathers."

At once, the skylark swooped down to investigate. The old man, noticing the bird's interest, beckoned her over and said, "Good morning, my young friend. And what can I do for you?" The skylark asked, "How much are the worms?" And the man responded, "Two for a feather, my child; and the coach is nearly full of them." The bird couldn't resist. Yanking out a small feather from underneath her wing, she dropped it into the man's hand and said, "Two, please."

And it went on that way for several days—the skylark having worms to her heart's content, sacrificing merely one feather each day. It seemed too good a deal to pass up. Until it wasn't. Over time, the little bird discovered she couldn't fly as she once did, and then the day came when she leaped up to join the other skylarks singing joyfully in the sky, only to fall flat on the ground instead. The consequences hit her with horror. Though she had grown plump on the worms, her wings, body, and tail had lost their lustrous cover and exposed spreading patches of bald skin.

She knew what she had to do—gather enough worms to buy back her feathers. She hopped and hopped until it felt as though her legs would fall off, hunting for worms and piling them up until she had all she could carry.

Exhausted and desperate, the skylark slowly hopped over to ask the man who had happily taken her feathers how many feathers he would give her for her collection of worms. The man peered at her closely, threw back his head, and laughed. He drove on down the road, shouting back over his shoulder, "Worms for feathers is my business, sonny; not feathers for worms!"

The story is summed up this way: "And the sorry end of it all was that the skylark lost his wings and the ability to fly and the desire to sing, and at last died, leaving nothing of him but a little heap of dust on the earth that he had exchanged for the blue sky of heaven."[7]

Addicts know exactly what happened to the skylark. They've experienced what it feels like to wake up one day and realize, far too late, that their chosen fix has taken them prisoner.

An addiction—either chemical or behavioral—is any mood-altering, compulsive behavior(s) we use to dull emotional, psychological, and spiritual pain born of the trauma and spiritual homelessness we ultimately can't kick despite negative consequences. Our addictions are fueled by the mistaken belief that something outside of us can heal the pain inside of us. In the next chapter, we'll look more closely at how addictions are the ego's way of trying to solve the universal problem of human suffering without relinquishing control and surrendering to God or a Power greater than ourselves.

The way an addiction starts and escalates can be outlined in five stages:

1. Step 1: Pain.
2. Step 2: The use of a mood-altering chemical substance

(like drugs or alcohol) or the adoption of a behavior (like watching porn, overeating, or compulsively exercising) to anesthetize and distract you from inner pain.

3. Step 3: Temporary numbing and relief. ("I'm a genius! No more pain!")
4. Step 4: Bad consequences. ("Oh, dear, what have I done?")
5. Step 5: Shame and guilt that lead to a fresh round of pain and self-loathing that bring us back to step 1.

Lather. Rinse. Repeat.

Sound familiar?

Ponder for a moment the wounds you've been running away from so you don't have to feel them again. What behaviors or substances are you using that are helping you avoid facing your problems instead of learning how to live with them? How are these addictive workarounds screwing up your life instead of helping you cope with your deepest and most frustrated longings? Do they really alleviate your emotional pain, self-loathing, long-held resentments, and stinging regrets? Do they quiet the cruel voice of that finger-wagging prosecutor who lives rent-free in your head?

Now, don't fib to me (and yourself). The answer is that your little and not-so-little (or private and not-so-private) addictions and self-defeating behaviors are self-escalating. That's how it works. Always.

Our addictions are wicked smart. They know that our hunger for home and for a cure for our psychological, spiritual, and emotional distress is bottomless. Psychiatrist and renowned addiction expert Gabor Maté likens the addicted parts of us to "hungry ghosts," ravished creatures who have "scrawny necks, small mouths, emaciated limbs, and large, bloated, empty bellies" who cope with their inner tumult by gorging themselves on anything that will fill the hole in their souls.[8] Unfortunately, they can't get enough down their skinny gullets and into their aching stomachs to satisfy themselves.

Right now, some of you already know you're chemical or behavioral addicts and that you need help. You can't stop smoking weed, rescuing your troubled kid (even when you know it's hurting you and her), blowing up at loved ones or colleagues, or eating to escape from your feelings. Perhaps you bought this book in the hope that it would help you find freedom. If this is you, read on.

Some of you, however, are still not convinced you're on the addiction continuum. You're uncertain whether one of your troubling repetitive behaviors(s) is an addiction or merely a peccadillo. Okay, let's clear that up. Have you ever set out to prove to yourself (and maybe others) that you're not powerless over something by limiting or abstaining from it for a specific period of time?

"I'll only gamble during football season."
"I'll only do weed edibles on Saturdays."
"No more hard liquor for me. I'll only drink beer or wine."
"I'll abstain from all social media for a year."
"If I'm successful, then I'll know I don't have a problem."

In my experience, people who aren't addicts don't set out to prove to themselves that they aren't. It simply doesn't occur to them.

Try this on. Have you ever felt the need to put controls in place to prevent yourself from doing something, like emptying the house of Chardonnay; putting a pornography blocker on your computer, phone, or tablet; or lining up a friend to call you every day to ask if you're doing something you no longer want to do?

And, finally, if you really want to know if you have a problem with something, then try this: just stop it.

If on your own willpower, you can stop overeating, lecturing your twentysomething kids on how to live their lives or make better decisions, playing Elden Ring until the wee hours of the morning, using nicotine (in any of its many forms), or working eighty-hour weeks ("I do it all for the kids!"), then God bless you. Give yourself a hug and buy yourself another worm.

On the other hand, if you hate a compulsive behavior but can't stop it, if you keep digging cisterns that don't hold water, then you're an emotionally and spiritually wounded addict who needs help. Don't feel bad. We're all desperate for a fix. There's simply no other way to be in this world as we know it.

A Recovery Story

Have you ever read C. S. Lewis's book *The Great Divorce*? It includes the perfect illustration of the journey from addiction to recovery. In it, there's a ghost of a man who has a reptile perched on his shoulder that whispers in his ear, saying he can't possibly live without him. Soon an angel appears and asks, "Shall I kill it?"

At this, the ghost desperately begins to make excuses for

why he can't live without the creature on his shoulder, even though he knows it's destroying him. "May I kill it?" the angel asks the ghost-man again. After many repeated—and rebuffed—efforts by the angel, eventually the man reluctantly gives his permission, and the angel slays the reptile. What happens next always chokes me up. The ghost metamorphoses into an actual man and the reptile becomes a magnificent white stallion, which the man mounts and joyfully rides away.[9]

This is the story of my recovery. Drugs, alcohol, and all my other addictions were like a reptile on my shoulder telling me I couldn't live without them. For a long time, I preferred to "be ruined rather than changed," as poet W. H. Auden wrote.[10] But when I hit bottom and gave my higher power consent to heal me, the reptile of my addiction transformed into a gift I could share with others rather than a curse. This can be the story of your recovery as well.

In the pages that follow, I will present the Twelve Steps as a spiritual solution for our spiritual homelessness, a program that will help you find sobriety and heal from the wounds of your past and the unhappy behaviors they supply with fuel in the present. I believe this design for living can teach you how to address your insatiable longing for God, for healing, for completion, and fulfillment. It won't necessarily fix *everything* that ails you (nothing can!), but it will teach you how to regard and untangle your problems in a completely different and spiritually healthy way. The Twelve Steps have saved the lives of millions of hopeless, spiritually bankrupt people who, when at their bottom, found themselves standing in front of the last house on the block with nowhere else to go. The Twelve Steps can do this for you as well.

One day, shortly after I arrived at the treatment center, I met with a counselor named Skye, who reminded me of the godmother of punk rock, Patti Smith. She was a diminutive woman in her sixties, with long, flowing red hair and wearing clothes that looked like she made them at home on a loom. She radiated so much empathy and kindness that the moment she walked into the room, I wanted to lay my head in her lap and snot-bubble cry like a baby. Skye invited me to share my story with her—what I was like before the hideous reptile of addiction perched itself on my shoulder, before the pain of unexamined trauma, childhood wounds, and my sense that I'd never fit in the world led me to use mood-altering substances and other addictions to cope with life.

When I finished rehearsing my tale, her eyes puddled, and she said something that changed the direction of my life. "I think you've endured enough already, don't you?" she asked, in a voice that I imagine sounded a great deal like the angel from *The Great Divorce*. I wept and said yes. Skye then told me something that blew me away. She said she had read the story of a woman, who was an early member of A.A., who said that the concept of *salvation* in the Bible has a secondary meaning that few people know about—it means "to come home."[11]

And so I ask you, haven't you endured enough already? Don't you want salvation so that you can—finally—come home?

Chapter Three

WITHOUT A PADDLE

In this short Life that only lasts an hour
How much—how little—is within our power.

Emily Dickinson, "In This Short Life"

STEP ONE

We admitted we were powerless over _____
—that our lives had become unmanageable.

The classic film *Monty Python and the Holy Grail* is a hilarious satire of the legend of King Arthur and the Knights of the Round Table, setting out on their mission from God to recover the Holy Grail.

In an iconic scene, King Arthur confronts the Black Knight, who is guarding a bridge that Arthur wants to cross. The defiant knight warns Arthur that anyone who tries to pass must die. Impressed with the Black Knight's confidence and bravery, Arthur invites him to join his Round Table, but the Black Knight refuses and insists on a fight.

Early in the battle, Arthur severs the Black Knight's left arm, and blood spurts everywhere. Despite the grave injury, the Black Knight refuses to surrender, saying, "'Tis but a scratch. I've had worse."

Next, Arthur cuts off the Black Knight's right arm, but he still won't give up. "Just a flesh wound," he argues, in his risible refusal to admit defeat.

Sighing, Arthur chops off the Black Knight's right and left legs. Now cut down to a torso, the Black Knight begrudgingly agrees to "call it a draw."

But as the King and his squire Patsy ride off, the Black Knight, now reduced to a limbless torso, continues to throw taunts at them. "Running away, eh?" he screams at Arthur. "You yellow bastard, Come back here and take what's coming to you. I'll bite your legs off!"[1]

Who wants to embark on a new way of life by admitting complete defeat? The first time I read Step One, I felt like lawyering up and sending God a cease-and-desist letter. "Powerless? Unmanageable? I think not, good sir!"

When we're kids, our hypercompetitive culture tells us losing is shameful. The important adults in our lives admonish us never to wave the white flag. *Fight to the bitter end!* If you don't believe me, just watch those foamy-mouthed fathers running up and down the sidelines at their eight-year-old's soccer game, yelling at their clearly miserable kid, "Win, Billy, win!"

Even when I eventually did warm up to my therapist Jamie at the treatment center, I still resented being told I was powerless over drugs and alcohol (not to mention my other addictions). Okay, I had a "willpower problem." But look, I hadn't lost my home, marriage, kids, health, or job because of my substance use. I mean, really.

Maybe you live in a handsome home in a tony gated community. You have a fat 401(k), and your kids get good grades and attend church youth group every week. By all appearances, you seem to be coping very well, thank you very much. How could your life be unmanageable?

Let's spend a little time on this question. Relax your arthritic grip on denial, just long enough to hear me out. Before we go any further, we have to get this right. Step One is the only Step you must do 100 percent perfectly, or you can't move on to the ones that follow. Honestly, working the Twelve Steps can be stupid hard, and you won't be motivated to do the work if you're not *absolutely convinced* you're out of ammo and your life is an unbridled mess (or trending swiftly in that direction). But once you are? Paradoxically, it becomes very, very good news.

My Life Is Unmanageable

The Twelve Steps teach that your life is, or eventually will become, unmanageable as the result of your addiction(s)—or simply as the result of being a vulnerable biped prancing around a planet hurtling through space at 67,000 miles per hour, take your pick).

I have friends who lost their marriages because of their porn addiction. I know people who lost their relationships with their children and suffered heart attacks as a result of their workaholism. I know gambling addicts who bet gazillions of dollars on the White Sox (at the time of this writing, a sure sign your life is unmanageable). I even know a model train enthusiast (a hobby I can't wrap my brain around, but whatever) who secretly bought twenty thousand dollars' worth of model freight train cars before his wife uncovered his secret credit card and demanded he begin attending Spenders Anonymous meetings. And the list goes on.

It's possible that your personal misadventures haven't (yet?) dragged you as far down the scale as these people. Maybe your story isn't as thrilling or tabloid-worthy as mine or others, but you might want to err on the side of caution.

After all, you wouldn't be meandering around the self-help aisle if a little part of you wasn't in pain and feeling confused, ashamed, fearful, and frustrated that, despite your best efforts, you can't do what you want to do or stop doing what you don't want to do.

For example, you might be taking a few too many anti-anxiety meds or nightly draining a bottle of wine while making mac and cheese for the kids, endlessly scrolling through TikTok, or eating compulsively to self-soothe. Perhaps you find yourself in familiar cycles of controlling or manipulating others to get them to do what you want, or seething with resentment because they didn't do what you want. Obsessively chasing success at the office to prove to yourself (or maybe your deceased mother) that you're worthy of love.

Now ask yourself, *If I'm managing my issues so well, why do I keep looking for the next fix?*

For me, unmanageability revealed itself in the amount of time I spent thinking about getting, taking, and concealing substances when I could have been thinking about my relationship with God, myself, and others. It revealed itself in the negative thoughts and feelings that consumed me because I hated myself for repeatedly succumbing to my self-destructive behaviors. Unmanageability appeared in my defensiveness and arguments with loved ones who expressed concern about my behavior. It appeared in feelings like shame, apartness, isolation, and being stuck.

You might not be ready to walk into a meeting and say, "Hi. My name is _____, and I'm an addict." I get it. It can take a while. You also may have lived a relatively charmed existence up to this point, or maybe you're fortunate enough to be crushing life right now. Your addictions aren't presently causing you enough pain that you feel willing or motivated to put in the effort to work a program as challenging as the Twelve Steps. This program is, after all, for broken crayons, not for folks who haven't gone through the wringer yet. If you think you're doing just fine, I suggest you put this book on the shelf until the day comes when you hit the wall and you're in enough pain that you'll do anything to get out of it. Though it sounds unkind, I hope that fateful day comes sooner than later. It'll save you time.

If you didn't just put the book down, let's keep going and explore what it means to be powerless.

I Am Powerless

The Twelve Steps don't say we're powerless over our *lives*. What we initially need to cop to is that we're powerless over our *addictions* or habitual *self-defeating behaviors*. We do wield a fair amount of agency in everyday life. We have the power to get out of bed in the morning, take our kids to school, and go to work. We even have the freedom and power to love our moocher brother Marty, even though he still hasn't paid us back for covering his rent ten years ago.

And we have the power to do a lot of damage when we refuse to admit our powerlessness over our addictions. If we don't feel at home in this world, if we compulsively keep doing stuff that hurts us and others to numb the pain of the present and the past, then we do not have the power to fix ourselves. Listen, how can any of us think we're powerful and in control of our lives when half of us can't sneeze without peeing our pants? I mean, seriously.

Once we start indulging our addictions, they take on a power in our lives we didn't know we were choosing to hand over to them. When I drink water, I can put it down once I've quenched my thirst. But if I throw back a shot of tequila, I'll soon buy a case of Jose Cuervo and lock myself in a hotel room for three days.

I can only maintain my sobriety by remembering my *powerlessness* over the first drink. The same is true of my addiction to attention and affirmation from the group, conflict avoidance, and Sara Lee Iced Orange Sheet Cake (chilled, please), among lots of other stuff. If I'm being completely honest, I don't have the power or self-discipline to stop these behaviors on my own once they leave the station. I don't have a record of knowing how to brake. I need help.

Here is the truth that Step One requires us to reconcile with: we need God, and we need a God-initiated solution to heal the wounds that are driving our addictions and all-too-predictable self-sabotaging behaviors.

What is it you're powerless to control or stop once you start? Is it viewing porn, trying to get your alcoholic partner or child to stop drinking, saying yes with a cheerful but weary smile to every request for help that comes your way, compulsively running from one romantic relationship or marriage to another, looking for someone to "complete" you?

Though the Twelve Steps don't come right out and say you're powerless over life, once you admit you're powerless over your addiction and enter a program of recovery, your eyes suddenly open, and you see you actually are *mostly powerless over everything in life.* The only alternative to this truth is to believe the lie that you can play God in controlling how your life plays out. Please, that's like believing you can tell your cat what to do. I mean, you can't . . .

Listen, life is bigger than you are. Reality wins 100 percent of the time. If you refuse to believe me on this one, you will become deeply resentful when life laughs at your self-created programs for happiness, indignant when people won't follow your wonderful plan for their lives, or utterly confused when your partner leaves you, despite your impassioned case for why they should stay.

Life does what life does to us. We can't successfully control or exercise power over people, places, circumstances, and things—only our response to them. We can refuse to believe this and try to boss the world around or cunningly charm it to do what we want, which only leads to our becoming psychiatric patients. Or we can learn how to work with life on life's terms. This is another gift of the Twelve Steps.

Ego, Not Amigo

Here's why it's so important to clarify what it means that our lives are unmanageable and we are powerless over our addictions: you come equipped with an inner persona who works hard to convince you that your life doesn't need fixing.

Meet your ego.

Your ego is that radically selfish, self-centered voice in your head that wants the world and everyone in it to organize their lives around your priorities. We all know that voice.

It's that entitled and narcissistic lunatic in your brain that gets really, really chippy when others don't recognize how special you are and don't drop everything to satisfy your every want and need. *Don't you know who* I think *I am?* our ego shouts.

In my recovery program, we say, "Your ego is not your amigo," a rather twee aphorism but wicked true. The Twelve Steps tell us that your tyrannical ego runs your life on self-will and self-propulsion. It bangs guardrail to guardrail through the world, plowing into everybody and everything, all the while telling you, *Don't worry, honey. I got this.*

Moreover, your ego really, really, really wants you to believe you have far more power and control over your life than you actually do. Your ego tells you you're the producer, director, and Oscar-worthy star in the ever-running soap opera titled *Your Life.*

Atta girl! Look at you, running the show! your ego whispers in your ear while you blow through your world like a Category Five hurricane.

Your ego will explain away or refuse to see whatever contradicts its wishes. It is the seat of sin in your life. *It wants you to believe you're God.*

This brings me to a big point. Countless spiritual teachers have taught that every human being is addicted to at least one thing (which a Twelve-Step program can help solve)—the disease of "wanting to play God," of wanting to subtly (or not so subtly) control and exercise dominion over everybody and everything. This is the core addiction, the one underlying all other addictions. The addiction to control is often hard to spot because you've been at it your entire life. It's always there.

People in my recovery program like to say, "There is a

God, and it's not you." So true, fortunately. If you think the world is a flaming fiasco now, imagine the lunatic asylum it would be if you or I actually *were* God. Twelve-Step work focuses much of its energy on ego deflation and healing us of our need to run everything.

According to Saint Paul, the Buddha, and many schools of psychology, someone has to die if you're going to get well—and that someone is your imperious ego. It's what Jesus meant when he said, "He who loses his life for my sake will find it" (Matthew 10:39 RSV). It's what Saint Francis meant when he said (in the prayer popularly attributed to him), "And it is in dying that we are born to eternal life." And it's what Paul meant when he said, "Indeed, I have been crucified with Christ. My ego is no longer central" (Galatians 2:20 MSG).

But your ego will not "go gentle into that good night."[2] It always has a skillet on the stove, cooking up another cocka-mamie plan for staying in charge. It knows that if you admit you're powerless and not in control of your life, that your life is unmanageable, then the ego will be exposed, and you'll see it for what it is—that false, small part of you that wants to continue governing your life from the shadows with your conscious or tacit consent, even though it's killing you. That's why your ego will do everything in its power to keep you trapped in denial.

The Twelve Steps will compassionately but pointedly puncture your ego and return it to its proper size, place, and function. The Steps will transform you back into a creature instead of a self-appointed creator. Ironically, this is a great relief. It's exhausting and scary playing God. This is a lifelong challenge because just when you think you've got your ego in check, you discover that the wily little devil backed itself up to the cloud when you weren't looking and is downloading itself back into your personality's operating system once again.

You Have a Superpower

Okay, so why is giving up playing God, admitting powerlessness, and acknowledging the unmanageability of life good news? The Twelve Steps begin by teaching us we can't sincerely begin the spiritual journey until we admit we're spiritually bankrupt and utterly defeated. This is the paradoxical, bottom-side-up calculus of the gospel as well. "For when I am weak, then I am strong," says Saint Paul (2 Corinthians 12:10).

And let's not forget what happened when Jesus embraced powerlessness and accepted seeming defeat on the cross. The result was a *eucatastrophe*—"a turn in fortune from a seemingly unconquerable situation to an unforeseen victory."[3]

It's good news because, as it turns out, powerlessness is a superpower. It's where the healing begins.

As Ernest Kurtz and Katherine Ketcham write in *The Spirituality of Imperfection*, "God comes through the 'wound': Our very imperfections—what religion labels our 'sins,' what therapy calls our 'sickness,' what philosophy terms our 'errors'—are precisely what bring us closer to the reality that no matter how hard we try to deny it, *we are not the ones in control here.* And this realization, inevitably and joyously, brings us closer to 'God.'"[4] And it's so easy to tap into this superpower. As my friend Kathy says, "All you need is to admit your need."

When my son Aidan was three years old, my wife charged me with giving him a bath. When I realized I didn't have a towel to dry him off, I quickly ran to the linen closet to get one. When I returned, however, I discovered Aidan had taken an epic poo in the tub. Honestly, it looked like the aftermath of the Exxon Valdez oil spill. I feared for the penguins and harp seals. From the look on Aidan's face, it was clear he knew he had caused a disaster as well. He had gotten poo all over his hands from trying to pick up little fecal buoys, which he then tried to clean off by wiping his hands on his hair, face, torso, and the tiled walls. The more he tried to clean himself, the worse things became.

Well, Dad to the rescue! Aidan had to give up trying to control things by trying to fix himself (which only made things worse!) and instead allow a higher power (me!) to step in and clean him up. He had to hit bottom (sorry) and let me rescue him. This is precisely where Step One aims to take us.

The importance of hitting bottom and admitting power-lessness is a supremely Christian idea. As A. W. Tozer wrote, "The reason why many are still troubled, still seeking, still making little forward progress is because they haven't yet come to the end of themselves. We're still trying to give orders, and interfering with God's work within us."[5]

In describing his own hitting bottom, Saint Paul wrote the words every addict cries out: "I do not understand my own actions. For I do not do what I want, but I do the very thing I hate. . . . I can will what is right, but I cannot do it. For I do not do the good I want, but the evil I do not want is what I do" (Romans 7:15, 18–19 RSV). Do you not hear the powerlessness and the feeling of life's unmanageability in those words?

I didn't learn Romans 7 in seminary as much as I did the night I suffered a seizure in a Los Angeles hotel room where I was staying while on a business trip and had tried and failed to quit taking Xanax cold turkey. Thankfully, I found half a bar of Xanax at the bottom of my briefcase that staved off my potentially lethal withdrawals while I frantically called my doctor to get him to prescribe me more to tide me over. That night, though, lying in a pool of sweat in my bed, I felt like I was trapped inside the chorus of a Hank Williams song. I told God I gave up. I couldn't go on like this. I'd used up my last "good idea," and I'd die if he didn't help me.

In that moment, the strangest, most beautiful thing happened. I felt my chest relax and dilate, and an overwhelming sense of relief washed over me, as if every atom in the room shimmered with the Presence. Paradoxically, once I gave up the delusion of power and control over my life, another Power flowed in, gently saying, *Don't worry, I got you.*

I'm told that when certain types of aircraft go into a "graveyard spiral," a beginner pilot's first instinct is to pull up on the controls, which is the worst thing a pilot can do. When you pull up on the controls during a graveyard spiral, the plane goes into a steeper, more violent dive. The trick to survival is to *let go of the controls,* and the plane will level itself out.

This is the message of Step One. When your ego feels out of control, it will instinctively grab the controls and double down on what doesn't work, sending you into a steeper descent. If you admit powerlessness and let go, God will save you.

And wouldn't that be a welcome relief.

Chapter Four

HELPLESSLY HOPING

Hope begins in the dark, the stubborn hope that if you just show up and try to do the right thing, the dawn will come.
Anne Lamott, *Bird by Bird*

STEP TWO

Came to believe that a Power greater than ourselves could restore us to sanity.

If you're anything like I was when I first worked through the Steps, you're feeling a little peevish right now. In Step One, you were told you were powerless over your addictions (oh, and people, places, and things) and that your life was unmanageable (I'm sorry, *what*?). And now, in Step Two, you're told you're insane.

When does the fun end, people?

But if you read Step Two carefully, you'll realize it offers you precisely what you need at this point in the journey—namely, *hope*. Yes, you're powerless, and your life's a bit (or a lot) janky, but you're *not* beyond help. In Step Two, you encounter a dazzling idea—there might be another way. Your life can change, and things can get better.

In this chapter, I will discuss what *coming to believe* and being *restored to sanity* mean and deal with that prickly topic of "a Power greater than ourselves" in the next chapter, where I'll focus on *turning our will and our lives over to the care of God as we understood him.*

Step Two reveals the spiritual nature of the Twelve Steps for the first time. Once you've completed Step One, your first question will likely be, "Okay, who's going to clean up this mess?" and Step Two says, "a Power greater than you." For some, this is welcome news, but for others . . . not so much.

For the spiritually skittish, the whole "God-thing" can be a bitter pill. I can't tell you how often I've sat in a Twelve-Step meeting and heard a newcomer angrily cry, "You scammed me! First, you got me to admit I'm screwed, and now you tell me I can't get unscrewed unless I believe in some cosmic delusion. I woulda dropped out of this program weeks ago if I'd known the God-train was coming."

If you're in this camp, please know I understand. You undoubtedly have many good reasons for not wanting anything to do with God, much less organized religion. Maybe you were raised in a militantly secular home where the snarky atheist Christopher Hitchens was revered, and believing in anything spiritual was evidence that you had suffered a very nasty bump to the head. Or worse yet, you're the hapless victim of an ill-conceived Christian homeschooling experiment that left you able to recite the Gospel of Matthew from memory but unable to perform basic math.

All kidding aside, though, countless people have tearfully shared with me heartbreaking stories about their giving up on God. Some were raised in fundamentalist churches that bludgeoned them with passages from the Bible about a God who relished smiting sinners who look a lot like them. As kids, they prayed for God to save a loved one's life or to rescue them from an abusive home, but he didn't show up, at least not like they asked him to. Others were told they weren't welcome in their church or even their family's home because something about them didn't conform to people's expectations.

Thankfully, the Twelve Steps offer a way forward, not only for people who want a proven tool for strengthening their spiritual life within their religious tradition, but also for those who have given up on the idea of God and the church, for people who have moved beyond the religion of their childhood, and for folks who have suffered spiritual trauma and are no longer sure if or what they believe.

Even the most cynical seeker will warm to the idea of believing in a higher power when they learn that Step Two doesn't say *"believed* that a Power greater than ourselves could restore us to sanity," but *"came to* believe that a Power greater than ourselves could restore us to sanity."

What I'm trying to say is that if all this "coming to believe in a higher power" or "God-talk" has you wrapped around the wagon axle, then take a breath, cowgirl. There's no rush to figure everything out. You can take your time. You don't have to swallow all of Step Two in one bite. This God, Ultimate Reality, Great Fact, Spirit of the Universe, or whatever you want to call him/her/it right now doesn't wear a watch. He has all the time in the world. I've been following Jesus for a long time, and I'm still "coming to believe." I pray the journey of discovering the Presence in all things will never end.

Bill Wilson wrote that "the Realm of Spirit is broad, roomy, all inclusive; never exclusive or forbidding to those who earnestly seek."[1] Phew! That should cheer you up as well. Believe it or not, you can take anything to be your higher Power for now. Honestly, your DOC (Divinity of Choice) could care less if you think it resembles Snoop Dogg or the actor Steve Buscemi. It won't mind if you call it Howard (as in "Howard be thy name") or Marge.

Your higher power won't ask you to shave your head, wear an orange sari, bang a tambourine, and hand out tracts to uninterested people at the airport to win its love and approval. Moreover, this divine Power doesn't want your money and won't ask you to lead the middle school youth group. It loves you so much that it will rush to your aid, even if all you do is sarcastically roll your eyes in its direction and limply beckon it, grumbling, "Okay, whatever." The only nonnegotiable is that *this ultimate power can't be you*. You're probably a reasonably decent person, but your track record proves you're a woefully deficient deity.

If you're a spiritual seeker, the only thing required of you in this Step is a *willingness* to believe there's something or someone bigger than you in the cosmos that can fix your particular brand of crazy. That's it! You don't have to believe anything specific about God right now. Only be *willing* to believe.

In fact, I encourage you to avoid getting too specific about the name or identity of your higher power for the time being, even if you're a Christian and think you already have it all buttoned up with Jesus. There's no telling what kind of weird conception of God your scheming, threatened ego will conjure up for you, if it hasn't already. Lord forbid that you might return to a terrible mental image of God, one you mistakenly adopted or were handed when you were a kid. For now, run with a stripped-down version of God. He won't mind.

In addition to willingness, Bill Wilson wrote that Step Two requires *openness*. Japanese Buddhists have a word—*shoshin*, which means "beginner's mind" and denotes an open, curious orientation toward the world. A person who practices beginner's mind is free from preconceptions and prejudices. They are free and present to observe and explore things as they are rather than through the lens of their preexisting biases.

The beginner's mind is playful, easily amazed and delighted, open to new possibilities and fresh insights into life. The person who has adopted the posture of a beginner's mind doesn't approach things with a fixed point of view but always asks, *To what new way of seeing the world do I need to avail myself?*

Not only did the Buddha say that the beginner's mind is important on the spiritual path, but Jesus did as well, only he would have called it "child's mind," as in "unless you return to square one and start over like children, you're not even going to get a look at the kingdom" (Matthew 18:3 MSG). We should adopt this mindset when we deconstruct and reconstruct our understanding of who God is, whether we identify as Christians or not.

Adopting a beginner's mind was tortuous for a guy like me who has two seminary degrees and presumed he knew much more about God than he actually did. And yet, laying down my preconceptions about God was precisely what I needed to do. I went through a turbulent season of deconstructing and reimagining my faith in my early thirties. Since then, however, I've learned this process isn't a one-and-done deal. The only thing I know for sure at this stage of my life is that *God is love* and that we are the object of his furious affection. After that, all my beliefs are provisional and open to constructive interrogation.

That's what happened to me in treatment. I went through a process of uncovering, discovering, and discarding many of my old ideas about God. Apparently, I had a bunch of them.

Otherwise, what was I doing on a ropes course with ten other middle-aged addicts and alcoholics trying to get sober again? Good grief.

"Coming to believe" means giving God consent to introduce himself to you. Trust me, strange and wonderful things will happen when you become *willing* (again, not convinced, certain, or committed yet) to entertain the notion that God exists and is eager to help you.

All this inclusive, woo-woo talk sounds a tad too loosey-goosey to Christians who are anxious for people to immediately designate Jesus as their higher power and be done with it. Here's where I might get crosswise with a few folks: I don't think God or Jesus cares whether you know their given names or not, especially in the beginning.

Listen, if I was walking down the road and happened upon a badly injured guy screaming at me, "Hey Dexter, help me!" do you think I'd look down my nose at him and say, "Not until you call me by the name on my birth certificate, champ." Heck no! The guy will bleed out if I don't help him right away. Maybe when he's back on his feet, I can tell him my name is Ian. Similarly, I don't believe Jesus would withhold aid from a struggling spiritual seeker just because she had no clue about the identity of the person she was crying out to for help. Jesus often appears to people in disguise.

And here's how I know Jesus frequently works incognito in people's lives. I've repeatedly seen miracles only God could have accomplished in the lives of agnostics and even atheists who initially chose the strangest things to be their higher power. For example, I know a guy now in recovery named Mark who wanted to believe in God but couldn't make the leap because he had been molested by his youth pastor when he was a kid. One day, his sponsor, Phil, became frustrated with Mark as they were meeting in the rehab dining room where Mark was a patient. "Look, I don't care who or what you make your higher power for the moment. Right now, the person in charge of your life—namely, you—is a maniac who's apparently hell-bent on destroying your life. Heck, for the time being, you could make that Coke machine over there your higher Power for all I care," Phil said, gesturing at the vending machine in the corner.

And so Mark made the Coke machine his higher power.

Laugh or scorn all you want, but that "Coke machine" changed Mark's life. In two years, he went from living in his car to having a wife, a steady-income job with benefits, and a nice home. A few years later, Mark swapped out the Coke machine for a more traditional expression of God (as some people do) and found a faith community that he and his wife currently participate in and enjoy. Mark incorporates his Twelve-Step program into his faith in a way that doesn't compromise either, and the result is wonderful.

I'm not saying this is what happens to everybody. But who am I to tell Jesus he can't show up and perform miracles in people's lives in the guise of a vending machine, at least for a little while? I know people who make their recovery group, nature, or art their higher Power. God isn't proud. As a friend once told me, "Love always stoops."

For Bill Wilson, everything came down to becoming a seeker. He once wrote, "We found that God does not make too hard terms with those who seek Him."[2] Don't those words sound familiar? "Ask and it will be given to you; seek and you will find; knock and the door will be opened to you. For *everyone* who asks receives; the one who seeks finds; and to the one who knocks, the door will be opened" (Matthew 7:7–8, emphasis added). The older I get, the less worried I am about who is "saved." I believe God opens the door and welcomes all genuine spiritual seekers home.

If you're a spiritual seeker, your work in Step Two is to open yourself up to the possibility of believing that a benevolent force exists in the universe that wants the best for your life. When you do (even a little), a seed will plant itself in your heart, and something that looks like faith will eventually sprout without your having to lift a finger. Thankfully, it's not the quantity but the quality of faith that matters on the recovery journey. And if you can't muster anything that resembles openness and willingness, then experiment with acting "as if" there's a Power greater than yourself that can restore you to sanity, and then see what happens. If you do, you will awaken one day to find you've crossed a meridian into a land of faith.

Now if you're someone who really resists the notion of God or simply can't imagine one, do what a friend of mine did with one of her sponsees. She had her write a personal ad for a higher power she could believe in. It read, "Single, newly sober woman looking for a loving and merciful God she can trust to be in charge of her life. This God must have infinite years of experience forgiving and guiding messed-up people. He should be kind, patient, faithful, and enjoy British television."

I have no idea if God watches the BBC, but I do know he's kind, patient, and faithful. He will gladly oblige if you ask him to reveal himself to you (as he eventually did for my friend's sponsee). Again, all you need is a thimbleful of *willingness*. God will take it from there.

Ironically, Step Two and the notion of "coming to believe" is often harder for Christians to complete than for spiritual seekers (as are Steps One and Three). The problem is they tend to breeze by these Steps, presuming, *I already completed these Steps when I gave my life to Christ.*

Well, maybe you did . . . or maybe you only sorta did.

When I came into the program, I realized that what I'd learned in Bible studies, during multiple seminary stints, and from years in church ministry was that my clerical-collared ego had often been in charge all along, gorging himself on theological knowledge and leadership training that I could use to maintain control of my life and author my own salvation. I had intellectualized rather than experienced God. I hadn't surrendered my life to Jesus as much as unwittingly tried to exploit Jesus to fuel my self-prescribed programs for happiness—namely, to win people's approval, to compensate for growing up in a screwed-up family, and to work out my family-of-origin issues through other people. I unconsciously wanted to rent his power to help me stay in control of my life and in the lives of others.

God quickly made it clear he wouldn't cosign that loan. While in treatment, I told my group therapy littermates that I'd spent a decade and stupid amounts of money earning two seminary degrees, that I had written popular books about the spiritual life and had spoken at large conferences around the world about the love and power of God. Following this shameless brag, a guy said, "Yep, and here you are."

Clearly, my old version of Christianity had ultimately failed me.

I also came to see that even though I was a Christian, my conception of my higher Power (who I choose to call God) was terribly confused and distorted, which made Step Two harder. As we all know, our first mental impressions of God are rooted in childhood and are based on how we see and experience our parents or early caretakers. I realized that even though I had been a Christian for years and had done a lot of therapy, my understanding of God was still largely based on my relationship with my parents, who were cold and distant.

I also had to rinse out the view of God my childhood church had given me. As a kid, I attended a strict Catholic church and parochial school that had shrewish nuns who convinced me God was a capricious, homicidal madman given to random acts of violence. I had to vanquish those and all the other nutty ideas I had about God.

But here's the good news: working the Second Step allows Christians and seekers alike to examine their old ideas about who God is and ask themselves if they're entirely true or if they need updating. Isn't it possible that you need to strip away your false ideas about God and refresh your mental images of him?

A Twelve-Step friend in Vermont told me a story that beautifully illustrates the importance of reviewing and amending our distorted or archaic beliefs about God. He had been in a meeting with a young, clean-cut kid named Matt, who had recently been busted for drunk driving. It was Matt's first meeting, and that night's discussion topic was about being open to believing in a Power greater than ourselves that could restore us to sanity. Matt sat quietly listening until the end of the meeting, when he sheepishly shared that he had been raised in a conservative Mormon sect but didn't think God wanted much to do with him anymore. "God's really angry and disappointed in me," Matt said, unable to raise his head. "My parents tell me he hates drunkenness, but I can't stop drinking. I'm doing everything I know how to do to regain his trust, but I keep failing."

When the meeting was over, my friend eavesdropped on a conversation between Matt and a veteran group member named Motorcycle Mike, who walked over to welcome him. Mike couldn't have been more different from Matt. Six-foot-four and skinny as a fence post, Mike had long, stringy black hair and wore a beat-up leather jacket and oil-stained jeans with a wallet chain dangling off his belt.

"Dude, your God sucks," Mike said, shaking Matt's hand.

"I'm not sure what you—," Matt said, thrown back on his heels.

"He sounds like one mean son of a bitch to me," Mike continued. "My God's compassionate and forgiving. He always gives people like us second chances. You wouldn't believe the things I did back when I was drinking and doing coke, but my God loves me anyway. Tell you what," Mike said, his eyes widening as though a light bulb had suddenly switched on over his head. "Why don't you borrow my God until you find a better one?"

I don't know how Matt responded, but I hope he took Mike up on his offer. Anything would've been better than his old, distorted conception of God.

The best way to begin Step Two, then, is to acknowledge that even though you're a Christian, maybe you don't know as much about God as you thought. There's a famous prayer in Twelve-Step circles called the "Set Aside Prayer" that perfectly captures the posture we should adopt as we approach Step Two: "God, today help me set aside everything I think I know about you, everything I think I know about myself, everything I think I know about others, and everything I think I know about my own recovery [my own life] so I may have an open mind and a new experience with all these things. Please help me see the truth."[3] That's the beginner's mindset I commend to everyone who wants to refine or update their understanding of God.

Finally, you won't get through Step Two until you accept that you're worthy of a relationship with this God who wants to restore you. It doesn't matter if you think you're an irredeemably deficient loser (which a lot of us secretly fear we are beneath the surface). As Archbishop Desmond Tutu once said, "God has a particularly soft spot for sinners. . . . There is hope for us all. God's standards are quite low."[4]

Copping to Your Insanity

Now to the second half of Step Two and the sticky matter of your iffy mental health. Initially, I was put off by the suggestion that I was insane. I had an uncle (may he rest in peace) who once climbed naked onto the roof of his home and announced to the neighbors that he was Napoleon Bonaparte. Now *that's* insane. I have no problem admitting I'm a little off-kilter, but I've never claimed to be an early-nineteenth-century French despot.

Thus, when I expressed discomfort with the term *insane*, Sponsor Steve reminded me of our program's definition of insanity: "Insanity is repeatedly doing the same thing and expecting different results." Yes, it's a tired, hackneyed trope, but there's a reason it's overused—*it's the freaking truth!* Go on, take an honest look at all your addictions and crazy looping cycles of self-defeating behavior that you keep repeating despite the fact that they don't serve you, even a little, and tell me you're not certifiably batty.

Seriously, how many more times will you sneak downstairs in the middle of the night to eat a pint of ice cream before you finally accept that it won't fix your pain? How many more times will you delete the search history on your browser to hide stuff you don't want your teenage son to accidentally discover on your computer? How many more relationships will you wreck because you keep trying to control people who can't stand your desperate efforts to tell them what to do? How long will your approval addiction prevent you from having reasonable boundaries and saying no every now and then? How long will you remain weirdly loyal to a relationship with someone who repeatedly breaks your heart and will clearly never change?

Few things demonstrate how nuts we are than the never-ending stream of crazy thoughts darting around our brains like giant schools of startled minnows. All human beings are addicted to their habitual and predictable patterns of crazy thinking. We attach and identify with our thoughts, and no matter how hard we try, we can't seem to change them, particularly those that hurt us. We assign meaning and value to these thoughts that they don't deserve. After a while, these thoughts become who we are rather than evanescent bubbles passing on the surface of the river of our consciousness. Research says that the average person thinks tens of thousands of thoughts every day.[5] For me, around nine thousand of them are wacky and on autoplay.

In *The Untethered Soul,* author Michael Singer suggests a thought exercise I found helpful.[6] Picture yourself spending a day with an actual person who spoke to you in the words of your inner monologue. Imagine you can't escape this person any more than you can elude your buggy stream of thinking. They are glued to your hip. And like the stream of thoughts in your mind, this person just won't shut up:

"Why can't you do anything right?"

"You'll never change."

"You're overweight and boring."

"You're a sorry excuse for a parent."

"Buy a new pair of shoes. That'll make you feel better."

How much time would you need to spend with this person before realizing they're insane and determined to wreck your life? Apparently, forever, because that's how long you've been putting up with listening to them. You have not only spent your entire life in conversation with this deranged person in your head, but you've also gone so far as to try to argue and reason with them. We can't shake them because we're addicted to our depressed, anxious, narcissistic, self-prosecuting ways of thinking. How's that working out?

Listen, when I let my brain off its leash, all it does is eat the garbage. Thankfully, the Steps taught me how to relate differently to the crazy person in my head. One day, I realized that working the Steps had dramatically slowed the stream of negative self-commentary that used to scroll across the screen of my brain like a cable news ticker. I no longer assume that just because I think something, it makes it true. I learned to watch my thoughts move through my mind and let them go without getting hooked by them.

Step Two says a Power greater than yourself can restore you to sanity. The word *sane* derives from the Latin *sanus*, which means "wholeness" or "health." First, a healthy and whole person will no longer believe that their drug or compulsive behavior of choice can take away their unresolved traumas or feelings of not-at-homeness in the world. Second, they will no longer assign importance to or take their crazy thoughts and feelings seriously.

It wasn't until I started going to meetings and listening to other people describe their bat-crap, nutty behavior and identified with it that I became convinced I too was insane. One of the things I love about attending Twelve-Step meetings is that not everybody shows up crazy on the same day. Instead, we take turns. At some meetings, I arrive feeling like a lunatic; other times, I'm doing okay so I can be there for my friends who are crazier that day than I am.

Not long ago, I was sitting at a stoplight on a busy street. Not a nanosecond after the light turned green, a young guy behind me in his souped-up Ford F-350 laid on his horn and threw his arms up in the air as if to say, *Move, ***hole!* When I responded in kind, the guy had the gall to flip me off and mouth, "Effing loser."

Maybe I was tired. Maybe I needed a snack. But in that moment, my easily offended ego concluded that this incivility demanded a swift response. I threw my car into park, tore off my seat belt, leaped out of my Subaru Outback (an intimidating ride if there ever was one), and charged the guy's truck on foot, yelling and shaking my fists at him.

"What were you thinking?" one might reasonably ask. I wasn't. Looking through his windshield, I could see that this man frequented the gym, while I am a five-foot-seven string bean whose upper arms are the size of the cardboard core at the center of a paper towel roll. But I had lost my mind. Thankfully, the man in the truck mockingly smiled, shook his head, and sped off around me.

When I got back behind the wheel, my wife, Anne, angrily reminded me that half the drivers in Tennessee carry a 9mm Glock in the glove compartment of their cars for encounters such as these. I admitted I could have handled the situation with more aplomb.

That night, I shared this story at a meeting, and the room erupted in howls of laughter. Multiple people shared about either having done or thought about doing the very same thing in the past. And I thought, *It's good to know I'm not alone.*

And so, dear friend, relax. You're not alone. We're all on the lunatic continuum. If you know someone who isn't a little crazy, you probably just don't know them well enough.

Chapter Five

SOMEBODY TAKE THE WHEEL

The moment of surrender is the moment you choose to lose control of your life, the split second of powerlessness where you trust that some kind of "higher power" better be in charge, because you certainly aren't.

Bono, *Surrender: 40 Songs, One Story*

STEP THREE

**Made a decision to turn our will and our lives over
to the care of God as we understood Him.**

When my kids were little, my wife, Anne, and I took them
to Newport Beach, California, for an oceanside vacation. One
afternoon, while the family ate lunch, I took a much-needed
break from parenting and went for a swim *sans enfants*.

Once I reached thirty feet from shore, I rolled onto my
back and began lazily doing the backstroke. I was impressed
with how fast I moved atop the gentle ocean swells. *Why
didn't I go out for my high school swim team?* I mused, feeling
rather chuffed with myself. To my dismay, I soon discovered
why I was zipping through the water like Olympian Michael
Phelps—I was in the grip of a powerful rip current that was
swiftly dragging me out to sea.

Realizing my perilous predicament, I panicked and pulled
the ultimate rookie move—I frantically tried to swim against
the current to get back to shore. But alas, the "rip" was too
strong. Then I tried waving my arms and yelling for help
to people on the beach, but no one looked in my direction.
Completely exhausted, I began picking hymns for my funeral
when I caught sight of a lifeguard running down the beach
parallel to the water, followed by a gaggle of morbidly curious

onlookers interested in seeing if I'd survive or not. I had been summarily dropped into an episode of *Baywatch.* "Don't fight the current. Let it carry you!" the lifeguard yelled repeatedly to me through cupped hands.

I remember thinking that this metaphysical-sounding advice wasn't particularly helpful, given how dire my situation was. *Who did this guy think he was, Deepak Chopra?* To my surprise, however, my personal David Hasselhoff was right. I surrendered to the current until it gradually weakened, allowing me to swim to shore.

Step Three is called the "Surrender Step" because it's about ceding control of one's life to the Divine Current, or as Twelve-Step practitioners call it, "Letting go and letting God." In fact, people describe the progression of the first three Steps as, "I can't [Step One], God can [Step Two], and I think I'll let him [Step Three]." If that's not the gospel in miniature, I don't know what is.

Step Three is the "turning point," as Bill Wilson called it, the keystone on which the rest of the Steps are stacked. If you can't successfully take Step Three, return to Step One and start again. Don't feel bad if this is what you have to do. Though it sounds counterintuitive, going backward in the spiritual life can often result in going forward. Besides, there's no point continuing doing the Steps until you wholeheartedly buy into Step Three.

Why? Step Three drives home to us that the Twelve Steps are not a self-help program. As my first sponsor in early sobriety said to me thirty-five years ago, "We are well past any conversation about *you* fixing *you.*" Your willpower alone is no match for your addictions, the vicissitudes of life, and the undertow your ego creates through its self-sabotaging behaviors. There's no un-messing your messed-up life apart from surrendering the director's chair to God and letting him run the show.

Sadly, people of faith often communicate mixed messages about who is responsible for what on the spiritual path. For example, when I was in high school and hearing the gospel for the first time, I remember being taught that the development of a godly character was dependent on grace, not personal effort. I was told that all I had to do was give my life to Jesus, and I'd be filled with the Holy Spirit and gradually transformed into the likeness of Christ. C'est fini! But then I went to church, where I heard a contradictory message. I'd hear the preacher proclaim, "It's all grace!" but the unspoken subtext was, "But keep working to earn God's love anyway!" Oh, why do we make things so difficult for ourselves?

When a person tells me they're "trying to be a Christian," I know they don't understand the gospel, and their sneaky little ego is still at the wheel. You've met spiritually effortful people before, right? They're working their rear ends off to be like Jesus. They're always exhausted and feeling like they're "never doing enough," that they're a disappointment to God, a spiritual poser, and they need to "shape up or else!" These are good people. They mean well. They're just wrong.

Listen, the gospel is so easy we make it hard. *It's not about reformation but transformation!* It's about *letting go.* I know of no better definition for the word *faith* than this—"Let go!"

For the purpose of illustration, let's talk about the parable of the prodigal son. Regardless of what someone believes about God, I've never met an addict whose eyes don't tear up a little when they read or listen to this passage from Scripture. It's the archetypal recovery story. In it, we have a kid who wants to play God and exercise total control over his own life. The parable doesn't say he was an addict, but dang, he sure acts like one. He's narcissistic, selfish, demanding, entitled, childish, willing to mortgage his future to gratify his desires in the present, a suck on his family's finances, and an all-around plonker.

But then we're told the younger son looks at the mess he made of his life and "comes to his senses." In other words, he hits bottom and admits he's powerless over his addictions and that his life is unmanageable. That's Step One! Then he comes to believe his father (God) could help him. Hello, Step Two! Then he turns and heads home. Voila! Step Three!

And here's a sidenote: folks don't often see him this way, but the elder son in the parable of the prodigal son is every bit as much an addict as his younger brother. Like many people, he's addicted to his warped thinking—his self-righteousness, jealousy, sense of moral superiority, self-pity, and resentment. He has a twisted mental picture of his father. He sees him as unfair, a withholder of love, and unappreciative of his efforts to be the good son. This kid will also have to "come to his senses" like his younger brother did. He needs to meet his father again for the first time too.

When we rely solely on our own unaided efforts to give up our addictions and change ourselves into the likeness of Christ, we oppose the gospel of grace. That's called reformation! Grace goes into action when we finally give up trying to save ourselves, when we turn our will and our life over to the care of God as we understand him and let the current of

Divine Love carry us. We surrender and trust. If you want to "do" something, try positioning yourself in that section of the river where the current of grace runs deepest and swiftest, and then lie on your back and relax. Paradoxically, when you finally muster the courage to say to yourself, *I give up; I can't do it*, you're given the power to do it. That's called transformation!

Now, look, this chapter is brief because I don't want to overcomplicate this Step. You could be on the verge of a watershed moment. Are you ready to let go and surrender your addiction(s) and self-limiting compulsions and turn your will and your life over to the care of God as you understand him? Are you finally prepared to say to God, *I give up. Take my will and my life. I'm willing to go to any length to find sobriety, freedom, peace, and wholeness.* If so, can I suggest you do so right now? You may understand precious little about God, but if you get on your knees and ask him to remove your obsession with alcohol, drugs, work, controlling codependent behaviors, a harmful relationship, sex, overeating, people-pleasing, sports betting, or whatever your thing is, *he will do it.*

Does this sound mawkish or a little too "tent revivalish" for a person with your impressive curriculum vitae and privileged standing in the community? Or perhaps you're the tough, self-reliant type who still thinks, *God only helps those who help themselves.* For goodness' sake, don't let your pride or ego prevent you from doing the one thing that may very well save your life. If you're unpracticed with prayer and you're worried about saying the wrong thing, you can always recite the Third Step prayer from *The Big Book*: "God, I offer myself to Thee—to build with me and to do with me as Thou wilt. Relieve me of the bondage of self that I may better do Thy will.

Take away my difficulties, that victory over them may bear witness to those I would help of Thy Power, Thy Love, and Thy Way of Life. May I do Thy will always!"[1]

There, you did it. That wasn't too bad, right?

Now don't be surprised if, when you take the Third Step, you experience the beginning of a spiritual awakening, not unlike the one Jacob had when he looked up from his pillow and said, "'Surely the LORD is in this place, and I was not aware of it.' He was afraid and said, 'How awesome is this place! This is none other than the house of God; this is the gate of heaven'" (Genesis 28:16–17).

When I completed my Third Step, my obsession with alcohol and prescription meds was expelled and the world gradually began to look and feel very different. I discovered that if I scratched the surface of anything in this life, I'd find the face of God. I became acutely aware that the world brims with grace. I heard the wind blowing through trees and the call of the song sparrow as if for the first time. Borrowing a line from the Benedictine monk Bede Griffiths, "I was no longer the centre of my life and therefore I could see God in everything."[2]

I also stopped mentally time-traveling into the past and future and started trusting God in the present in a profoundly new and deeper way. Looking back, I had always viewed and experienced God as being far, far away, like a satellite circling the earth. I radioed my prayers skyward at him, hoping he would receive the transmission and then direct his answer back toward me or toward whomever or whatever it was that I was praying for. When I took the Third Step, I realized this distantiated vision of God was a horrible misunderstanding on my part. To borrow a phrase from Saint Augustine, God is "closer to us than we are to ourselves."[3] He resided in me all along. He was "the Great Reality deep down within us."[4]

For some, this felt experience of awakening is dramatic and sudden. For most people, it happens gradually over time. Here's how you can know if you've had a spiritual awakening:

> When a man or a woman has a spiritual awakening, the most important meaning of it is that he has now become able to do, feel, and believe that which he could not do before on his unaided strength and resources alone. He has been granted a gift which amounts to a new state of consciousness and being. He has been set on a path which tells him he is really going somewhere, that life is not a dead end, not something to be endured or mastered. In a very real sense he has been transformed, because he has laid hold of a source of strength which, in one way or another, he had hitherto denied himself. He finds himself in possession of a degree of honesty, tolerance, unselfishness, peace of mind, and love of which he had thought himself quite incapable.[5]

Does it sound too good to be true? Trust me, I know countless people whose doctors and families had given up on them who had the courage to take this Step and were set free from the snare of their addictions. Like Lazarus, they were brought back from the land of the dead. The Steps are designed to facilitate this experience, and Step Three is the great leap into the love of God.

Here's what Step Three looked like for me. Several months after I returned home from treatment, my wife, Anne, and I traveled to Encinitas, California, for a much-needed vacation. Every morning, I strolled along Cardiff State Beach, wondering whether or not the God I had believed in my whole life was worth believing in anymore. Clearly, my well-established idea of who he was had proven inadequate. I needed a new understanding and experience of God, one I could confidently "turn my will and my life over to." To make the point, I picked up a stone and addressed it as if it were Jesus. "Jesus," I said, "I need to let go of my old ideas about who you are before I can open myself up to receiving new ones from you." And with that, I threw the stone into the ocean as far as I could. Then I picked up another stone as a symbol of my still unformed conception and relationship with God and said the Third Step Prayer from *The Big Book*.

I suspect no one on the beach that day thought twice when they saw a middle-aged man ambling along the shore having a tearful conversation with a rock. I mean, it's California, right? But to this day, I carry that stone in my pocket. For me, it marks my entrance into the house of God, the gate of heaven.

Chapter Six

HUG THE CACTUS

Not everything that is faced can be changed; but nothing can be changed until it is faced.
James Baldwin, "As Much Truth as One Can Bear"

STEP FOUR

Made a searching and fearless moral inventory of ourselves.

People cock their heads to the side like a Golden Retriever that can't quite understand what their owner is saying when I tell them my spiritual hero is Pinocchio. I understand. Even *I* think it's odd that I've chosen a cartoon character to be my polestar.

In the Disney film version of this classic tale, the puppet Pinocchio leaves the home of his woodcarving creator, Geppetto, to embark on a quest to become a "real boy." But the kid barely even makes it to the end of the driveway before he falls in with a passel of ne'er-do-wells who convince him to become a sideshow act in a sketchy puppet show.

It's an inauspicious start to life.

Pinocchio soon becomes a celeb—and a money and fame-addicted celeb, at that. It's not long before things go sideways. Stromboli, the sleazy owner of the puppet show, imprisons his cash cow Pinocchio to prevent him from leaving his employ. Thankfully, Pinocchio's friend, the Blue Fairy, rescues him, and he vows to her that moving forward, he'll behave.

Alas. Pinocchio is cute, but he sucks at keeping promises.

At the suggestion of his criminally minded confreres, Pinocchio goes to Pleasure Island for a little "puppet self-care," to recover from his traumatic experience in Stromboli's caravan. There he parties like a Ritalin-fueled college freshman on his first fall break in Miami. He drinks and smokes like it's his job, gets into fights, smashes windows, and takes up playing pool and gambling. Clearly, puppet boy needs a good butt whoopin'—and life is about to oblige.

When Pinocchio discovers that the island hides a conspiracy to turn naughty boys into asses (something Pinocchio was already doing an excellent job of on his own) and sell them into slavery, he makes a run for it, narrowly escaping disaster again.

Now things take a Jungian turn. Pinocchio learns that while Geppetto was searching for him, his heartsick maker has been swallowed by the terrifying Monstro the whale. Determined to save Geppetto, Pinocchio descends into the cold and murky ocean depths and sneaks his way into Monstro's belly.

Of course, Monstro is an archetypal figure. His belly represents Pinocchio's shadow, that inky place inside himself where he must go to confront his psychological and spiritual bankruptcy, a step he must take before he can become a "real boy." Self-honesty—that's the price of admission to awakening, friends.

At the risk of his own life, Pinocchio rescues Geppetto and becomes a real boy as the natural consequence of facing his selfishness, self-seeking, dishonesty, self-centeredness, and indifference to the effect his actions have on others. He dies to himself.

Pinocchio's story is our story, at least mine anyway. We're flung into the world as unfinished and naive puppets longing to become real, but, unbeknownst to us, our ego is a maniacal puppeteer "pulling the strings" of our swollen instincts without our knowing it, inspiring us to do things that not only screw up our own lives but also the lives of others.

Like Pinocchio, we embark on our little (and not-so-little) moral misadventures until the day comes when we hit rock bottom and our souls summon us to enter our shadow (that part of our psyche where we unconsciously banish all those parts of ourselves we deem unacceptable) in order to confront, grieve, and integrate our darkness and make peace with ourselves. That Pinocchio successfully completes this journey and becomes fully human is what makes him my champion. And so Steps Four and Five are all about entering the belly of our own Monstro to face our own moral corruption, reclaim our "hidden wholeness,"[1] as Thomas Merton calls it, and become real men and women.

But this journey of self-discovery and spiritual awakening isn't easy. Personally, I avoided Step Four like I owed it rent money. When Sponsor Steve asked me when we were going to meet to go over this Step, I told him I couldn't finish it because I had radon poisoning. He wasn't amused.

But it makes sense, right? Who wants to enter their shadow to "make a searching and fearless inventory" of themselves? From the time we were in diapers, our ego has shone the light of our attention onto anything but our shadow. Wouldn't it be better to find a less demanding alternative, to remain blissfully asleep in denial's warm bed?

Trust me, my stomach turned when Sponsor Steve told me that working Step Four would inevitably involve facing the old ghosts that drove my addictions and cut me off from the "sunlight of the Spirit."[2] Lord, how dreary it all sounded. That said, I know that most people settle for as much spiritual transformation as will let them get by. I didn't want to be that person anymore, nor do I think you do.

Steps One and Two require little more than self-reflection. Step Three requires us to make a decision to turn our will and our lives over to the care of God, which is technically an "action," but not a particularly strenuous one, at least not for people who are desperate. When we arrive at Step Four, everything changes. Our lives are under new management. It's time to uncover, discover, and discard all the junk fueling our addictions. It's time, in the picturesque words of Mel Gibson, to stiffen the spine and "hug the cactus."

On October 14, 2011, Robert Downey Jr. invited Mel Gibson to present him with the American Cinematheque Award in Los Angeles. In his speech, Downey made these extraordinary comments about Gibson:

> When I couldn't get sober, he told me not to give up hope, and he urged me to find my faith. It didn't have to be his or anyone else's as long as it was rooted in forgiveness. . . . If I accepted responsibility for my wrongdoings and if I embraced that part of my soul that was ugly—"hugging the cactus," he calls it—he said that if I "hugged the cactus" long enough, I'd become a man of some humility and that my life would take on a new meaning. And I did, and it worked.[3]

And hugging the cactus will work for you too. This is the first of the "roll up your sleeves and brace yourself for some serious effort" Steps. No more abstract theological conversations about the "Great Uncaused Cause of the Universe."

The time has come for us to swim into Monstro's belly to exhume and examine our self-centeredness, grudges, character flaws, overindulged instincts, and our insistence on playing God and ruling the universe like an ill-tempered toddler.

In other words, like Pinocchio, we have to plunge into our pitchy waters to face the stark facts about ourselves and repent. I know, I know, I've just used another loaded term that conjures up horrid memories of "fireside chats" at church camp. But the word *repent* doesn't mean "crucify yourself for being a naughty boy or girl." For our purposes, let's define *repentance* as simply having a good long think about the lies we've told ourselves for far too long concerning what will make us truly happy, and what it has cost us and others. Like the prodigal son, the goal is to "come to our senses" and allow God to help us change our manner of thinking and living.

Step Four will prove difficult if you're dedicated to not finding out very much about yourself. My friend Mike once said, "The shortest distance between you and the person you want to become is the truth." Dang, if I don't sometimes hate the truth, especially when it's holding up a mirror to my fallen condition. But our sobriety and the healing of our lives depend on unflinching honesty with ourselves.

Thankfully, there's a sizable payday. Yes, our hearts will surely break in the process of working on Step Four (repeatedly, I'm afraid), but when they do, love, mercy, and forgiveness will fall into them through the cracks, I promise.

"Okay, how do I begin my Fourth Step?" you ask. Buckle up.

First, there is no single, universally agreed-upon format for making a "fearless and moral inventory of ourselves."

I've heard a million different ways to work Step Four. For our purposes, let's break it down into making three inventories or lists: Resentment Inventory, Fear Inventory, and Sex Conduct Inventory. Two additional helpful inventories—Harms Done Inventory and Skeletons in the Closet Inventory—are included in the workbook. We will be returning to these lists in Steps Five through Nine, so we need to do as thorough a job on them as possible.

Resentment Inventory

We begin by examining our lives through the lens of our resentments and long-standing anger. Why? Bill Wilson says, "Resentment is the 'number one' offender. It destroys more alcoholics [addicts] than anything else."[4] A person mired in resentment has little chance of recovering from their addictions. But what is a resentment? It is a feeling of "bitter indignation at having been treated unfairly."[5] It is emotionally reliving a past injury as if it were repeatedly happening in the present moment. Human beings are Velcro for resentments. We start picking them up from the moment we pop out of the womb, and, tragically, most people take truckloads with them to the grave.

Let's be frank, shall we? Most of us are unaware of how many grievances we're harboring and the role that unresolved anger plays in our lives. We're mostly out of touch with how furious and resentful we feel toward ourselves for not being able to live up to our ideals and toward our difficult life circumstances over which we seem to have scant control—the anger we feel toward the people, places, things, and institutions that regularly hurt or disappoint(ed) us, and yes, even toward the God who invited us to this party. Most of us worry that if we were to go into that room in our hearts marked "Anger," we'd burn up and disintegrate the same way a satellite does when it reenters earth's atmosphere.

Now listen, I know that coming clean about our deep-seated resentments isn't easy or pleasant. Most of us will do anything, even crazy self-harmful things, to avoid facing our anger. But we won't find healing and freedom until we make our "darkness conscious."[6] It's hard, but together we can do this. If we don't, Scripture tells us we will suffer.

The Bible is chock-full of examples of the negative consequences of holding on to old grievances. Cain felt so much resentment toward his brother Abel that he murdered him (Genesis 4). Leah held a grudge against Rachel because Jacob loved her more, which no doubt caused all manner of family problems around the holiday table (Genesis 29). And, of course, religious leaders resented Jesus for claiming to be the Son of God (e.g., John 5; 8; 10), and we know how that story ends.

Resentment and brushed-aside anger will corrode your life, which is why Jesus addresses it directly: "This is how I want you to conduct yourself in these matters. If you enter your place of worship and, about to make an offering, you suddenly remember a grudge a friend has against you, abandon your offering, leave immediately, go to this friend and make things right. Then and only then, come back and work things out with God" (Matthew 5:23–24 MSG).

I have a former friend who badly betrayed me. For years, when this person's name came to mind, my blood boiled, and I felt like choking the cat. Countless nights I lay in bed awake and fantasized about the butt kicking I wanted to give this guy for the suffering he had caused me. While sitting at traffic lights, I mentally rehearsed the scorching rebuke I'd one day give him, forgetting to notice that the light turned green until the person behind me leaned on their horn. Of course, this imagined showdown will never happen. Turns out, the guy has been dead for more than ten years.

"How long are you gonna carry that corpse around?" Sponsor Steve asked me when I shared this festering grudge with him. Steve is an honest guy—sometimes a little too honest for my taste, but he's rarely wrong. I grieve that I didn't let go of that resentment earlier and make things right with that old friend. It would have made both our lives easier.

All to say, resentments are like burrs in a sheepdog's coat—they're stupid hard to get out once they get entangled in your heart. But remove them we must! Our resentments and the anger that simmers right below the waterline of our consciousness threaten our newfound sobriety and cause more problems and spiritual unhappiness for us and others than we can fathom. Grudges are cancerous. As Elizabeth Gilbert writes, "As smoking is to the lungs, so is resentment to the soul; even one puff of it is bad for you."[7]

So as I began Step Four, Sponsor Steve instructed me to think back over the whole of my life and catalog the names of *every* person, place, object, institution, situation, or principle that had *ever* wounded or offended me. Then he told me to create a four-column diagram and put the names of the offenders with whom I had a resentment in the first column on the left and what they did to cause my resentment next to their name in the second column. (You can find the template for your Resentment Inventory in the workbook.)

Lots of interesting people and things made my resentment list. My second-grade teacher, Sister Mary Aquinas, excoriated me in front of my classmates for not knowing how to spell the word *colander* (why it was so urgent for a first grader to know how to spell the name of a common kitchen utensil still confounds me). I set down the name of my seventh-grade girlfriend Amy, who hooked up with my best friend Keenan, who, as a consequence of his hormone-driven betrayal, also made it into the Top Twenty on my grudge list.

My resentment list also included nearly every member of the past and current legislative, executive, and judicial branches of the US government; our neighbor's basset hound Digger, who bit me without cause when I was nine; climate change deniers; the names of every grade-school bully who ever gave me a wedgie (that list was surprisingly long); pastors who smugly believe they have a corner on the truth market; and the very snippy Nebraska state trooper who gave me a three-hundred-dollar-speeding ticket in 1987 for driving a mere 40 miles per hour over the posted speed limit. Honestly, how could he?

Of course, the names of the people toward whom I held a resentment in column 1 and the record of what they did in column 2 ran the gamut from these relatively minor offenses to the far more personal and painful wounds. The more serious perpetrators on my list included my abusive alcoholic father who broke my heart; my inscrutable mother who refused to leave him, even though she witnessed the ways he daily wounded her children; and a former employee who turned many longtime friends of mine against me after I let that employee go (with a *very* generous compensation package, I might add).

The point is not to leave anyone or anything off your grudge list—the trivial or the terrible. It doesn't matter if these people, places, ideas, institutions, principles, objects, or situations committed a misdemeanor or a felony against you—write down their names. Throw caution to the wind! Like Jackson Pollock hurling paint onto a canvas, fling onto the page the name of everyone and everything that has ever hacked you off—even a little.

Personally, I went way down the rabbit hole on this assignment. By the time I finished my Fourth Step inventory, I had a fifteen-page document with the names of forty-three offenders on my list. When I proudly showed it to Sponsor Steve, he said, "Take a break from writing your list for a few days and ask God to bring anything or anyone you might have forgotten to mind." A week later, I returned to him with a twenty-five-page document with many more names on my list.

What you'll notice when you're finished with your Resentment Inventory is that human beings can and do inflict a lot of pain on others. Some of the things people have done to you are dreadful. That said, you can't afford to allow your anger and resentments to hold you hostage anymore. They will suffocate you if you don't let them go.

Now, in the third column, we set down how the behaviors of these people affected us. To simplify the assignment, Bill Wilson gives us a few boxes we can tick if we like.[8] Did this person's behavior toward you bruise your *pride*? Check the pride box. Did their actions damage your *self-esteem*, interfere with your *personal relationships*, threaten your *material or emotional security*, interfere with your sex relations, or block your *social or professional ambitions*? Okay, check whichever of those boxes that apply.

You can work down your list this way or you can play with the format a little. As I've said, there's no one right way to do any of the Steps. For example, you can add more category boxes. But perhaps, like me, merely checking a box won't cut it for you. I'm a writer, by golly, and if there's a story to be told, I'm going to tell it . . . in color.

So Sponsor Steve told me to forget about ticking the boxes and instead write out in the third column as detailed an account as I wanted of what happened that led to my feelings of resentment, and to include not only the areas of my life the offense affected but also how it made me feel and the negative impact it had on my development as a person.

For example, when writing about a boyhood experience of sexual abuse, I couldn't just check off boxes. That painful episode demanded more unpacking and exploration. I wrote about the shame and rage I had to work through, and how it had led to my lifelong fear of emotional intimacy. Contrastingly, I didn't write three pages about Sister Mary Aquinas and her obsession with cookware. My resentment toward her wasn't so great that it required me to do anything more than tick a few boxes. That I gave scant attention to Sister Mary's unkindness gave me no small amount of satisfaction.

Now here comes the part of Step Four that initially made me so angry I wanted to throat punch Winnie the Pooh. In column 4, we're asked to reflect on and write down the role we played in the episode that led to our resentment. In almost every case, *The Big Book* says, we had a part.[9] What were our mistakes, faults, or character defects that played even a minor role in the creation of our resentment? Where was I self-seeking? Where had I been dishonest? Where had I acted out of fear, jealousy, or spite? Where was I at fault?

The suggestion that I was partly to blame for my sexual abuse or that I had done something that contributed to my father's alcoholism or that I deserved my colleagues' unjust treatment initially outraged me. Wasn't this victim blaming? Hadn't I already spent decades shaming and punishing myself for things I ultimately wasn't responsible for? And yet, the Twelve Steps teach that we always had some part to play in whatever happened that led to our resentments, even if it's miniscule or after the fact. Strangely, this is good news. If someone else is completely to blame, then you are a prisoner of their misdeed and have no power to remediate it. If you can see and own your part—no matter how minor that part might be—you have the jurisdiction and agency to do something about it.

For example, though I was not in any way to blame for my sexual abuse, I could reflect and come to see that I had later organized my self-concept around that terrible episode. I had believed that what had happened to me as a kid made me who I was as an adult. For years, I had unconsciously played the victim card. Honestly, it hurt when I recognized that I played a part in that miserable affair, *albeit after the fact*. That said, I could now stop using that experience as an excuse for not fully showing up for my life. What a blessed relief!

As for the work colleague I let go, I saw that they left shooting their six-gun over their shoulder at me because I had been a woefully inadequate manager. Seriously, Michael Scott from *The Office* has better managerial skills than I do. I had let them go before giving them reasonable opportunity to improve their performance. Though they had no excuse for trashing my reputation, I helped create the circumstances in which their behavior was understandable. Yep, I played a part in it.

As uncomfortable as it may feel, looking at our part in things is essential. You see, the ego convinces us that we're never to blame, or even partially to blame, for hardly anything that goes awry in our lives. It would rather we point the finger at anyone but ourselves. And yet Jesus tells us, "First get rid of the log in your own eye; then you will see well enough to deal with the speck in your friend's eye" (Matthew 7:5 NLT). That's solid advice. We become far more likely to forgive those who hurt us and let their offenses go when we accept that we played a role in what went wrong in our relationship.

On a sidenote, don't be surprised if a lot of old, painful memories and feelings come up for you as you work on this Step. Sponsor Steve explained to me that when we're in our active addiction, it's like we're in a car driving 100 mph down a windy road at night without our headlights on. Then, when we give up our numbing substance or compulsive behavior, it's like someone slams on the brakes, and all the emotional trash in the backseat comes hurling into the front seat—all our now unmedicated shame, fear, pain, resentments, and mental pictures of our stroppy Aunt Hazel. Furthermore, in the process of identifying our role in all that has gone wrong in our lives, we will also begin to see our character flaws in high-def, many of them for the first time. It's a lot to take in at the beginning.

The only way I know how to let go of resentments is to see my offender and myself through God-given new eyes. *The Big Book* tells us that when we look at our list, we'll see that we've allowed people, places, and things to dominate us.[10] We need to adopt a different way of being in the world. Here's how Bill Wilson suggests we view the people who hurt us:

> This was our course: We realized that the people who wronged us were perhaps spiritually sick. Though we did not like their symptoms and the way these disturbed us, they, like ourselves, were sick too. We asked God to help us show them the same tolerance, pity, and patience that we would cheerfully grant a sick friend. When a person offended we said to ourselves, "This is a sick man. How can I be helpful to him? God save me from being angry. Thy will be done." We avoid retaliation or argument. We wouldn't treat sick people that way. If we do, we destroy our chance of being helpful. We cannot be helpful to all people, but at least God will show us how to take a kindly and tolerant view of each and every one.[11]

As you can imagine I held a lot of resentment against my father. The list of his wrongdoings was long. As I followed the wisdom of the Steps and used time-proven spiritual practices that can bring about inner healing, my heart began to slowly warm toward my father, because these words in *The Big Book* perfectly described my father's problem:

> Those who do not recover are people who cannot or will not completely give themselves to this simple program,

usually men and women who are constitutionally incapable of being honest with themselves. There are such unfortunates. They are not at fault; they seem to have been born that way. They are naturally incapable of grasping and developing a manner of living which demands rigorous honesty. Their chances are less than average.[12]

The Steps helped me see that no one at the outset of their lives thinks to themselves, *I'd like to grow up to suffer from grave emotional and mental disorders that prevent me from being honest with myself.* No one thinks, *I want to hurt my wife and kids, not be able to hold down a job for long periods of time, and die at age sixty-two from alcoholism and drug addiction. What fun!*

Long after my father's death, his psychiatrist told me he had diagnosed him with narcissistic personality disorder and major depressive disorder. It all made sense. My dad had a very painful childhood. His mother was deeply troubled, which severely affected him and his siblings. My dad wasn't consulted about the challenges he would face in life. I'm not giving the guy a pass for unkind behavior; I'm just saying the Steps taught me that I have to take these facts into consideration when I evaluate my father's life and how his actions affected me.

While I was writing this book, my ninety-five-year-old mother died peacefully in her sleep. My mom was a force of nature. She was the kind of person who could smoke in a hospital and no one would stop her. She was loud and hilariously entertaining at parties, but nurturing children wasn't her strong suit. As one of my siblings once said, "We had Lucille Bluth from *Arrested Development* for a mother." Fans of *Arrested*

Development will know that the mother, Lucille Bluth, is wildly funny, but a little acerbic. That was my mom.

For years, I held a lot of resentment toward my mother. It wasn't until I completed my Fourth and Fifth Steps and began practicing spiritual disciplines designed to help foster forgiveness (more on this practice soon) that God gave me empathy, compassion, and love for the mother I had, and peace about the mother I didn't have. Prior to working the Fourth Step, I tried every remedy to help myself move on from my "mom issues," and many of them were useful. But it was working the Twelve Steps that helped me finally get the ball over the goal line.

But forgiving my mother and father while working the Fourth Step was only the beginning. Not long ago I was sharing an old resentment with my friend Patrick, a fellow recovering alcoholic, and he said something that nearly knocked me over: "What if you just forgave everyone?" he said casually, as if it was the most obvious and natural thing in the world to do.

"*Everyone*?" I asked, incredulously.

"Why not?" Patrick said, shrugging. "Issue a pardon and let 'em all out of jail!"

The idea that I had the power and freedom to forgive everybody who had ever hurt me in this life in one fell swoop blew my mind. I'm a priest, a therapist, and a spiritual director. Why the heck had I never thought of that before? And so later that day, I went to a secluded spot in my favorite park in Nashville, and peering out over the gentle rolling hills surrounding the city, I announced to God and the world that I forgave everybody for everything, including God and myself. Immediately I felt a great release. For me, this was one of the many gifts of working the Fourth Step.

"God?" you might ask. Yes, God would appreciate your understanding and forgiveness as well. We could have a long and heated theological conversation about the sinlessness and moral perfection of God and how presumptuous it is to think that he requires our forgiveness. Please, listen to me: Your emotions didn't go to seminary. Your anger and disappointment in God couldn't care less about your well-laid-out theological arguments. If even a tiny part of you feels disappointed or angry with God, you have to acknowledge it and work through it with him. Thankfully, he's a kind and patient listener.

Fear Inventory

Now comes that part of the Fourth Step that turned out to be the most valuable one for me—the Fear Inventory. *The Big Book* says that unresolved resentments and anger are the greatest threats to our newfound recovery,[13] but trust me, our conscious and unconscious fears run a close second. I had no idea how much fear ruled my life until I did my Fourth Step Fear Inventory.

Behind my generally confident facade, I'm afraid of failure, success, loss of reputation, bullies, people leaving me, financial insecurity, interpersonal conflict, something bad happening to my wife and kids, intimacy, rejection, being advised by my doctor to wear knee-high compression socks, and death, among other real or perceived threats to my well-being.

The problem with fear isn't simply that it's a sucky feeling; it's that it activates the very character flaws we'd most like God to remove from our lives. I promise you, fear skulks in the shadows of our grosser behaviors. When I brag about my accomplishments, it's because I'm afraid you won't like me unless I'm a big deal. When I procrastinate, it's because I'm afraid I won't do something perfectly from the outset. When I inappropriately blow up at one of my kids for doing something I think is dangerous, it's because I'm fearful they'll get hurt.

The Big Book says that when we are afraid, it's because "self-reliance failed us."[14] When we're frightened, it's often because we're trying to manage life on our own. Doing my own Fear Inventory was a revelation. I felt like I was seeing what was behind most of my problems and addictions for the first time—namely, terror! I also saw that surrender and God-reliance could provide the solution.

In column 1, write down all the people, places, principles, institutions, ideas, and objects you're afraid of, and then how your fear affects you in column 2. In the process of doing your Fear Inventory, you will also begin to identify false beliefs that produce anxiety, which you've been carrying with you throughout your life.

"If anything goes wrong in a relationship, it must be
     my fault."
"Bad things always happen to me."
"I'm not brave enough to try new things."
"I'll never get out from under the curse of my addictions."
"I always end up alone."
"I can't be okay unless everyone else is okay."
"People won't love me unless I'm a success."
"No matter how hard I try, I never do anything right."
"Change is too hard."

Identifying and writing down your fears and your false, anxiety-producing beliefs is the first step on your journey toward overcoming them.

Sexual Conduct Inventory

Okay, let's talk about inventorying our sexual conduct, shall we? Sadly, this is a topic fraught with countless differing opinions. One thing I hope we can agree on is that God created us as sexual creatures who naturally long for emotional, spiritual, and physical intimacy. Our sexual natures and powers are God-given and good. We should neither deny nor feel ashamed of them. That said, we know that when our sexual instinct and conduct run amok, they can cause disproportionate suffering and harm to ourselves and others.

Now listen, I'm not the arbiter of anyone's sex life. I'm not interested in wading into any controversies about what's okay and not okay. Frankly, that's not my business—that's between you and God. The fact is that we all have sex problems, right? And all of us have made mistakes in this area of our lives that spiritually and emotionally haunt us.

In *The Big Book*, Bill Wilson suggests we review and inventory our sexual conduct over the years and ask ourselves, *Where have I been selfish, dishonest, or inconsiderate? Whom have I hurt? Did I unjustifiably arouse jealousy, suspicion or bitterness? Where was I at fault? What should I have done instead?*[15]

You can use a graph to work on your Sex Conduct Inventory:

Column 1—**Whom did I hurt?** List of all the people you have harmed sexually.

Column 2—**The cause.** Be specific as to how your sexual conduct harmed the people on your list. Ask, *Where was I at fault? Where had I been selfish, manipulative, dishonest, or inconsiderate? Did I unjustifiably arouse jealousy, suspicion, or bitterness?*

Column 3—**What should I have done instead?** Specifically, what should you have done differently in each situation?

Remember, the point of this exercise is not merely to disburden yourself of guilt and shame. Ultimately, this exercise will help you work with God to identify your values and mold your ideals for your future sex life. When you've completed the inventory, spend time praying and asking God what he desires for you in this domain of your life moving forward.

* * *

Now as you put pen to paper, be aware that a full spectrum of emotions will arise while writing your Fourth Step. You will probably feel relief, regret, the joy of unburdening yourself, shame, sadness, anger, a heaviness of heart, a lightness of being, or perhaps all the above.

Listen, all these feelings are normal, and they will pass. The important thing to remember as you do the work is that you stand under the eternal, loving, non-blaming gaze of God. Though it might be hard to believe right now, you're going to look back on the experience of your inaugural Fourth Step with untold wonder and gratitude as you come to see that God was performing a mighty work in your heart while you were working this Step. Frederick Buechner sums up what you can hope for when you're done:

> The sad things that happened long ago will always remain part of who we are just as the glad and gracious things will too, but instead of being a burden of guilt, recrimination, and regret that make us constantly stumble as we go, even the saddest things can become, once we have made peace with them, a source of wisdom and strength for the journey that still lies ahead. It is through memory that we are able to reclaim much of our lives that we have long since written off by finding that in everything that has happened to us over the years God was offering us possibilities of new life and healing which, though we may have missed them at the time, we can still choose and be brought to life by and healed by all these years later.[16]

Now, don't dawdle. Pick up your pen and get to work.

Chapter Seven

FESS UP

There is no greater agony than bearing an untold story inside you.
Maya Angelou, *I Know Why the Caged Bird Sings*

STEP FIVE
Admitted to God, to ourselves, and to another human being the exact nature of our wrongs.

I once attended a Twelve-Step speaker meeting in a stately white Congregational church in southern Connecticut. Twelve-Step groups offer different meeting formats. In a speaker's meeting, one person stands at the front of the room and shares their story—what their life was like before and while they were using, and the "experience, strength, and hope" they're finding through the program and working the Steps.[1] These are powerful gatherings, especially when the speaker has never told their story publicly. I know from experience that laying bare the gritty details of your life before a group of strangers requires incalculable courage. I don't know of a more vulnerable exercise.

That night, a newly sober young woman named Janet (not her real name) shared her recovery journey with a sizable group for the first time. I've heard lots of painful "shares" in speaker meetings, but Janet's story was hard to listen to. She recounted growing up in poverty with two drug-addicted parents who trafficked her to support their meth habits. She described her own slide into drug and alcohol addiction, living in rat-infested hotels, selling her body in return for drugs and alcohol, neglecting and then losing her children to the foster care system, and more. Honestly, just when you thought her tale couldn't get any more tragic, Janet would reveal another even more shocking and heartbreaking detail.

At the end of a speaker's presentation, people usually respond with raucous applause and whistles, offer words of encouragement, and remark on places where they resonate with the speaker's story. That night, however, the story was so devastating and woeful that the group was brought to silence. It was a worse-than-awkward moment. Here was this emotionally naked woman standing in front of two hundred staring, open-mouthed alcoholics and addicts, waiting for them to say or do something—anything—but the only sound in the room was the hum of an overhead fluorescent light.

Thankfully, there was an old-timer at this meeting named Joanie, an outspoken eighty-five-year-old heiress with a tremorous voice who had forty-five years in the program. She was part of the first wave of A.A. members and a personal friend of Bill Wilson. She was universally loved among locals in recovery for her bluntness and wisdom. Joanie knew exactly how to respond in this moment. "The word of the Lord," Joanie said, creakily rising to her feet and clapping her hands in a gesture of reverence and respect for Janet.

"Thanks be to God," the rest of us whispered from force of habit, rising one by one to our feet to join Joanie's applause until the sound of clapping and cheers were nearly deafening. This wave of love and admiration washed over Janet, who wept with gratitude, relief, and joy while a large clutch of women spontaneously enveloped her in a group embrace.

We all have a story, and no matter how difficult, humiliating, or gut-wrenching parts of the story may be, it is sacred. Our life stories demand and deserve a full-throated sharing, not only for the sake of our own healing, but for the healing of the world that bears witness to their telling as well. Step Five is this act of "sacred telling."

If you think Step Four was hard, Step Five is harder. (I told you this wouldn't be a walk in the park.) For many, Step Five feels like an inconceivable lift. It was difficult enough to "make a searching and fearless moral inventory of ourselves" in Step Four, but now we are told we have to bare our souls and admit "the exact nature of our wrongs" to God, ourselves, and another human being. Honestly, we can't skip this Step in the process. "As long as you keep secrets and suppress information, you are fundamentally at war with yourself," writes Bessel van der Kolk in *The Body Keeps the Score*,[2] and he's right. If we want to emerge from our isolation and finally be free of the underlying causes and conditions of our addictions and compulsive behaviors, we have to tell someone "the all of it," as my Northern Irish friend Declan likes to say.

None of us would choose to do this on our own initiative. But as Sponsor Steve likes to remind me, "There's nothing the program will ask you to do that you were about to do right before you got here." Boy, is that true.

Furthermore, the Twelve Steps instruct us we can hold nothing back, no matter how frightening or embarrassing it might feel. We must face the fact that we teem with contradictions, that we are busted *and* beautiful. We are, after all, on a search-and-rescue mission to recover our true selves.

Your greatest enemy in this Step is your insecure, high-strung ego, which, with each successive Step, is losing its tyrannical stranglehold on your life and becoming increasingly desperate to remain in charge.

It will tell you that if you take Step Five, you will be exposed for the monster you are. You will be abandoned and cast aside by God and your fellows. Heck, if you take this Step, you'll be showered with shame! But I beg you from the outset not to kowtow to your fear. It's worth it! If you do this Step, you will join the millions of people who have experienced liberation from their past because they unreservedly worked it. I'm grateful to be counted among them.

One of the more important gifts of Step Five is that it will help you overcome the sense of aloneness you have felt for years. I've never met a human being who, to one degree or another, didn't suffer from the feeling of radical apartness that Adam and Eve dragged with them into the world when they exited the garden.

Keith Miller calls the Fifth Step "spiritual dialysis."[3] It's a spiritual exercise that helps flush guilt, shame, and loneliness out of our system. It's the spiritual equivalent of a week in detox.

If you've done a thorough Fourth Step, you now possess a record of your resentments, fears, mistaken beliefs, and sexual conduct. Now it's time to fully bring everything into the light of day with the Fifth Step by first meeting and sharing your story (1) with God, (2) yourself, and, finally, (3) another human being. When you've completed these three exercises, you will have an opportunity to reflect on and rejoice in the miracle of your accomplishment!

Admitted to God

I felt relieved that the first stop on my Fifth-Step journey was with God. I knew God wasn't going to gasp with surprise and feel faint when I confessed to him that time in my twenties when I got soused on the Lower East Side of Manhattan and forgot where I parked my car . . . for two days. As the author of Job writes, "His eyes are on the ways of mortals; he sees their every step" (Job 34:21). God doesn't miss a trick, friends. There's no point in hiding anything. It also makes sense that we should admit our failures to God before we do so with ourselves or another human being. Though we don't often think about it this way, God's heart grieves more than anyone's when we wound ourselves or others. Thus we owe it to him to meet with him first.

Because God knows everything there is to know about our inner worlds and personal histories, it's tempting just to gloss over this first stage of the Step. *God, you already know about my faults and the unfortunate things I've done, so there's no point in boring you with the details. Let's just say I'm really, really sorry for being a putz, and I'll try to be a better citizen in the future. Cheers!*

This kind of avoidant flyby simply won't do. No, we must be intentional and thorough when we meet with God to do our Fifth Step. On the day I did mine, I went to my church early in the morning when I knew no one would be there, placed two chairs on the altar facing each other (one for me and one for God), lit a candle, and placed it on the floor between them, and read my Fourth Step inventories out loud to God as if he were sitting directly across from me.

I imagined looking straight into his eyes and told him everything—and I mean *everything*. I never once said, "Aw, no need to tell you how much I resent my father. Surely you've read my bestselling memoir about my relationship with him." Thanks, but no thanks, ego.

No, I spilled the beans to God like he was a sympathetic, doe-eyed monk duct-taped to the seat next to me on a twelve-hour flight to Buenos Aires. When I finished, I felt closer to myself and God than ever before. While driving home, I reflected on an episode with my then eight-year-old son Aidan that helped me give language to what I had just experienced.

One Sunday afternoon, I was in our living room doing ab crunches on a big elastic stability ball when Aidan came in and asked me if I wanted to go outside and play catch. His face fell when I told him he'd have to wait until I was finished trying to transform myself into someone who looked less like the *Star Wars* character Jabba the Hutt.

A few minutes later, I stepped away from my workout to take a phone call in my office. When I returned to finish my exercise routine, I was shocked to find my stability ball lying flat and deflated on the floor with a hole in it. I didn't need the team from the TV show *CSI* to pinpoint the culprit in this homicide, nor to uncover their motive.

"Aidan!" I called out.

"Yes, Dad," Aidan said sheepishly, walking into the room.

"Did you pop my exercise ball?" I said icily, pointing to the blue rubber corpse lying at my feet.

"No," he said innocently. "Maybe it was Maddie."

This kid was digging himself a crater. Maddie is Aidan's big sister; she wasn't even home when said crime occurred. But rather than drag him into the interview room and force a confession from him, I told him I believed him and gently reminded him of how important it was to always tell the truth. I then let him go back outside to play.

Then I waited.

Not five minutes later, I was lying down reading on the living room couch when Aidan burst through the front door and collapsed in my arms. "Dad, I stabbed your medicine ball with a pen," he cried, burying his tear-drenched face in my chest. "I'm sorry, I'm sorry, I'm sorry," he said over and over again through a knotted-up throat.

Ironically, I never loved Aidan more than I did at that precise moment. As far as I was concerned, his confession was a formality. I had already forgiven him. When he admitted he'd made a mess of things, cried for what he'd done, and asked for my forgiveness, my heart immediately gentled toward him, and I wanted nothing more than to pardon and embrace him.

I've done some brainless stuff. But of one thing I'm sure— this is the posture God adopts toward us. He's always poised to forgive. Two thousand years after Jesus told the parable of the prodigal, God still throws his dignity aside and runs through the fields to sweep us into his arms before we even have a chance to utter the words, "I'm sorry." Many say they begin to feel this experience of mercy and divine welcome when they complete this first stop on the journey of their Fifth Step. I know I did. It is a mighty big Step on the path toward a spiritual awakening.

Admitted to Ourselves

So, this might sound strange, but I did my Fifth Step with myself while looking in the mirror. It was a completely different experience than writing it down or voicing my confession to God. When I looked myself in the eyes and enumerated my wrongs *out loud*, I felt the weight of what I had done, which I could now endure, having felt the mercy of God when I finished my Fifth Step with him.

Now it's time to admit to ourselves the exact nature of our wrongs. What does "exact nature" mean? It means examining our hidden motives, interrogating our mistaken beliefs, and trying our best to discern what caused us to commit specific wrongs.

For instance, I founded and worked at a church for ten years. As an entrepreneurial spirit, I should have handed the reins to a more managerial-minded person at year five, but I didn't. I hung in there and tried to be someone I wasn't, nearly bringing down the house I built. Those last years were rough for me, my staff, and my leadership. At times I was a mercurial, whiny martyr.

For years, I told myself that I stayed and suffered through those last five years because I was "a loyal and long-suffering Christian." There may have been a tiny element of truth to that, but while doing my Fifth Step, I realized I also hung on because I was a codependent, conflict-avoidant, approval seeker who was so terrified of disappointing others that I was willing to do anything (like staying in a job for waaaay longer than I should have) because I didn't want to let people down. It was a painful realization that rightsized my ego, but that's the point!

All that said, I also realized that my fear of disappointing others was born of a painful childhood experience of abandonment and the fear that people would hate and desert me if I left the pastorate. This offered me a countervailing dose of self-compassion.

The point is that if we want to be free, we have to lovingly confront and integrate our shadow. When my oldest child, Cail, was five years old, they went through a phase when they believed a giant monster living in their closet would come out and kidnap them while Mom and Dad were in bed down the hallway. Unable to sleep, Cail would crawl into our bed, waking Anne and me up multiple times a night. If you have kids, you know behavior like this will eventually make sleep-deprived parents secretly wish there really *was* a giant monster in their kid's closet that would ferret them away.

Eventually, I came up with a solution. One night, I sat on Cail's bed and told them that when they were ready, we would invite the big monster to come out of the closet to have a chat with us. When Cail gave me permission, I opened the closet door and asked the monster to join us. Acting as an interpreter, I told Cail the monster's name was Henry. As it turned out, Henry the Monster was lonely and wanted Cail to be his friend. As we spoke, Henry shrank in size until he was no bigger than one of the stuffed animals that lay beside Cail in bed. By now, Cail was relieved and all too happy to befriend Henry, who had become small enough to sleep beside them, and our problem was solved. The point is that our monsters and the shame they carry for us tend to shrink in size or sometimes even disappear when we let them out of our closet and talk with them.

Admitted to Another Human Being

I've had numerous people get all defensive and "Bible-quotey" on me when I espouse the benefits of admitting the exact nature of their wrongs to another person. They usually say something like, "I don't need to confess my sins to anyone except God. Only he has the authority to forgive!" As a therapist, I understand this unconscious resistance to the idea of sharing our wrongdoings and failures with another person. It's a terrifying prospect.

Now listen, I am by nature a private person. I cringe when people overshare, particularly on social media. Seriously, don't you ever wince when someone divulges a heavy, deeply personal struggle on Instagram? Does the whole world need to know that information? No! That said, Sponsor Steve says, "Not *everybody* needs to know everything about you, but *somebody* does."

Few things are as liberating as when we confess our moral failures and long-held dark secrets to another person and they don't run from the room, hand covering their mouth, making that whooping sound our dog makes right before it throws up.

Nor will Scripture let us off the hook on this matter. Bill Wilson studied verse 16 of chapter 5 in the epistle of James before he wrote this Step: "So confess your sins to one another, and pray for one another, and this will cure you" (5:16, paraphrased). Apparently, James (and Bill) was keyed into the idea that "you're only as sick as your secrets" long before present-day therapists.

James implies that if we don't reveal the truth about who we are (both the bad and the good!) to somebody, we risk remaining in isolation and suffering the burden of carrying harmful secrets. Obviously, the person listening to your Fifth Step doesn't have the authority to forgive you. That's way above their pay grade. What they can do is give you what in my tradition is termed an "assurance of pardon." In my experience, James is right. My Fifth Step relieved me of my guilt, shame, and loneliness. It opened the door to a deeper spiritual awakening in my life.

One of the many gifts I also received from sharing my Fifth Step with another person was perspective. For as long as I could remember, I felt like I was irredeemably deficient, that I lacked something important that everyone else had and that rendered me unworthy of love and relationship. Alternatively, there were times when I felt I was head and shoulders above everyone else. I was caught in the cycle of either being a "hero" or a "zero." I ping-ponged back and forth between these opposing poles so often that I should be permanently wearing a neck brace for whiplash. That all changed when I finished sharing my Fifth Step.

My sponsor told me about things he'd done that made me realize I wasn't nearly as bad as I thought, nor as awesome as I believed. I was shocked and relieved to learn that other people had made the same mistakes I had. For the first time in my life, I felt the joy of being just another "bozo on the bus" of life—no better and no worse than anyone else. Of course, once you grasp this, it will be an affront to your narcissistic ego, which relishes the feeling that it is either the "best of the best" or the "worst of the worst."

An additional perk of sharing my Fifth Step with another human being was the discovery that I was forgivable. Do you know what it's like to tell another person all the weird stuff you've thought, felt, or done—stuff you've been terrified to share with anyone—and have them not reject you? I even remember moments when my sponsor and I laughed at a few of the ridiculous things I had done, especially when he shared similar stories from his own experience. What a relief!

Guidelines and Tips

First and foremost, you must choose the right person to hear your Fifth Step. Whoever you choose must be 100 percent trustworthy. They must understand their sacred duty to take your Fifth Step to their graves without ever breaching your confidentiality. Is it possible you might pick the wrong person, who will gossip about what you shared with them in your Fifth Step? Yup. But I've been around Twelve-Step groups for thirty-five years, and I've never once heard of this happening.

I encourage you to do this Step with your sponsor or another person in recovery who has done their own Fifth Step. It's essential that this person knows how difficult and important it will be for you to take this Step. It's also vital that this person be willing and sufficiently discerning to give you honest feedback, point out your blind spots, or gently call you out when you're ducking something that needs naming.

In my experience, broken people make the best confessors. Personally, I look for someone I know who has experienced enough suffering and personal failure in their own life that nothing I say will shock them. In other words, I want a confessor who has "history." Lord knows I don't want to share my weird and twisted inner world with someone whose life resembles a Thomas Kinkade print. I want someone who will be as open with me about their struggles and wrongdoings as I am with them about mine.

If you don't have a sponsor, you can share your Fifth Step with your therapist, clergyperson, spiritual director, or a highly trusted friend, preferably one who has known you for a long time. I've included a set of instructions in the workbook you can share with the person you ask to hear your Fifth Step if they've never done it before. It outlines the Fifth Step's purpose, the person's specific role, and what they should and shouldn't do.

Regarding scheduling, I prefer to do the Fifth Step in a single session, which, in my case, took several hours. (I've heard of some that lasted a full day, but that's for overachievers.) A single session might be too exhausting or emotionally overwhelming for some folks. No worries. There are no set rules or one right way to do this. If a single session isn't possible or desirable, break it into two or three sessions, preferably scheduled close together. It's normal to want to put off doing your Fifth Step with excuses such as, "My inventory isn't perfect," but know that this won't be the last time you make a Fifth Step. It's better to do a mediocre Fifth Step the first time around than not to do one at all.

So, make an appointment with your listener as soon as you finish your Fourth Step. Make sure you choose a quiet place where you won't be overheard, interrupted, or stared at should you get teary (which you probably will).

It's tempting when reading your Fifth Step to give in to one of three errors—self-justification, depression, or self-contempt, the latter being my NOC (neurosis of choice). Self-justification sounds like this: "I purposely abandoned my annoying ten-year-old little brother Jimmy at a Mobil station in South Bend for six hours, which may or may not have traumatized him. But the pesky little jerk deserved it, right?" Uh-uh. That's not a confession; that's whitewashing.

And then there's lapsing into maudlin self-introspection. I learned about this during one of my Fifth Steps with my friend Damian, a Reformed theologian and Jungian analyst with a PhD in bluntness. At the beginning of our meeting, I told him I thought I was the worst sinner in the world. "Oh, you're much worse than that," he responded. Damian knew my self-flagellation was merely a bid for his pity and words of reassurance. *That'll teach you not to go fishing for sympathy,* I thought.

When a person tells me all the terrible things they've done and claims that they're probably unforgivable, I tell them not to flatter themselves—I know plenty of people who are *way* worse than they are. I also remind them that many of the world's most notorious sinners eventually became our most revered saints. Take the probable sex addict Saint Augustine of Hippo, for example. I dare you to fool around and carouse like he did. Well, not literally.

Prior to his conversion, Augustine spilt more beer than Keith Richards ever drank. Canonized in 1303, he was made patron saint of brewers by the Catholic Church. No fooling. Look it up. Then there's Saint Mary of Egypt, who prior to her conversion allegedly coupled with anything that wasn't secured to the floor. The point is that the greatest of sinners often have so overwhelming an experience of forgiveness and grace that they become the greatest of saints. This could be you!

When I do the Fifth Step, I begin by reciting this marvelous prayer from Anglican bishop George Appleton:

> Give me a candle of the Spirit, O God, as I go down into the depths of my own being. Show me the hidden things, the creatures of my dreams, the storehouse of forgotten memories and hurts. Take me down to the spring of my life, and tell me my nature and my name. Give me freedom to grow, so that I may become my true self, the seed of which You planted in me at my making. Out of the depths I cry to You.[4]

And then I take Bill Wilson's advice from *The Big Book*: "We pocket our pride and go to it, illuminating every twist of character, every dark cranny of the past."[5]

I encourage you first to share the scariest, most humiliating, and shameful items on your Resentment, Fear, and Sexual Conduct inventories rather than put them off until the very end. It's much easier if you get these out of the way right out of the gate. Now listen, I had what was, or what felt like, pretty shameful stuff on my list, but I've learned from doing my Fourth and Fifth Steps that sin is uncreative and predictable to the point of being boring.

I challenge you to come up with a new and novel transgression that no one before you has ever committed. Hopefully, you'll discover this when the person listening to your Fifth Step periodically interrupts to tell you they've done the same things you've done (or perhaps something even worse).

The point is, you won't feel alone anymore; the old loneliness and feeling of apartness will disappear. You won't feel like your particular brand of busted is special or unique.

Now begin with the four columns on your Fourth Step Resentment Inventory list—who you resent, why you resent them, how it affected you, and what part you played. For me, this was a profoundly difficult but healing exercise. For the first time in my life, I recounted how my experience of sexual abuse prevented me from having deep relationships. I began to see the false stories I had told myself about myself and about the way I thought the world worked.

I uncovered broken lines of code in my heart's programming. I exhumed the mistaken belief that I was a worthless misfit who God thought was a pest. I finally saw through the lie that if people really knew me, they'd be repulsed. I saw the lie I'd told myself for years—that people would never love me for who I am, so I needed to project a false self to win their love and approval. And here's a biggie: I finally realized that alcohol, drugs, and my other addictions were not my *problem* but only the *symptom* of my problem. Substances and process addictions were my misguided and disorganized solutions to the pain and problems that came from the lies I told myself.

Johann Hari, the author of *Chasing the Scream: The First and Last Days of the War on Drugs*, writes, "I was taught by the people I met—and by the growing scientific evidence—that we are all more vulnerable to addiction now because we are increasingly isolated from each other, and from the things that give us meaning. As I say in the book, *the opposite of addiction isn't sobriety; it is connection.*"[6]

Loneliness and disconnection are endemic in the contemporary world. Surely you have experienced their bitter taste at some point in your life. This was one of the big problems that fueled my addictions. I have a big group of friends. Lots of people listen to my podcast and read my books. And yet I didn't feel truly connected to anyone, including myself. I knew them but failed to connect with most of them at the deepest level. I found a connection among my Twelve-Step recovery friends. Let's be honest—most of us are lonely. Few things will kill the human spirit like disconnection. What Step Five does is relieve us of the belief that we are separate from God, ourselves, and others.

Finally, if you stick with the Twelve Steps as a design for living, you will do many Fifth Steps over the years. It's good spiritual hygiene. Period.

When You're Done with Step Five

My friend Larry had terrible arthritis in his hip but for years refused surgery because he had a phobia of going under anesthesia and was afraid of postsurgery pain. Finally, when the pain in Larry's hip became infinitely worse than his fear of surgery, Larry went under the knife. When I spoke to Larry a week after his surgery, he was ecstatic. "I had no idea how much pain I was suffering and how negative an effect it had on my quality of life until I didn't have it anymore," he said. "I wish I had done this years ago. I would have enjoyed life more."

Larry's story perfectly illustrates what happens once you have your Fifth Step behind you. Once released from the burdens of your secrets, resentments, shame, and guilt, you realize just how much pain you've been in for years and how much better your spiritual quality of life would have been had you done it sooner. For years we lived in what teacher Tara Brach calls "the trance of unworthiness,"[7] that voice in your head that repeatedly tells you, *You're not enough; you'll never be enough.* For me, the litany of negative self-talk quieted significantly after my Fifth Step.

The Big Book describes how we might feel after we take the Fifth Step: "Once we have taken this step, withholding nothing, we are delighted. We can look the world in the eye. We can be alone at perfect peace and ease. Our fears fall from us. We begin to feel the nearness of our Creator. We may have had certain spiritual beliefs, but now we begin to have a spiritual experience. The feeling that the drink problem [or whatever problem] has disappeared will often come strongly. We feel we are on the Broad Highway, walking hand in hand with the Spirit of the Universe."[8]

Do not be surprised if you encounter grace in a startling new way following your Fifth Step. Theologian Paul Tillich captures the experience perfectly in *The Shaking of the Foundations*:

[Grace] strikes us when, year after year, the longed-for perfection of life does not appear, when the old compulsions reign within us as they have for decades, when despair destroys all joy and courage. Sometimes at that moment a wave of light breaks into our darkness, and it is as though a voice were saying: "You are accepted. *You are accepted*, accepted by that which is greater than you, and the name of which you do not know; perhaps you will find it later. Do not try to do anything now; perhaps later you will do much. Do not seek for anything; do not perform anything; do not intend anything. *Simply accept the fact that you are accepted!"* If that happens to us, we experience grace. After such an experience, we may not be better than before, and we may not believe more than before. But everything is transformed. In that moment, grace conquers sin, and reconciliation bridges the gulf of estrangement. And nothing is demanded of this experience—no religious or moral or intellectual presupposition, nothing but *acceptance.*[9]

May you finally know the joy of divine acceptance.

Chapter Eight

OKAY, I'M WILLING ALREADY

"Do you want to be healed?"
Jesus of Nazareth (John 5:6 RSV)

STEP SIX
Were entirely ready to have God remove all these defects of character.

STEP SEVEN
Humbly asked Him to remove our shortcomings.

There's an often-told parable among people in A.A. about a group of Twelve-Step folk embarking from a pier to motor out to Serenity Island. Just as they pulled up anchor and floated away, a few of them at the stern caught sight of one of their A.A. friends running out onto the pier to join them. One of them was upset that "Mary" had missed the boat. But another one called out to her, "Mary, jump into the water and swim—we'll pull you up with us!"

They saw Mary plunge in and begin swimming steadily toward them. At first they thought she was going to make it—she had a good rhythm going. Then, suddenly, they saw her struggling to stay afloat. "Mary, drop the rock!" they shouted.

Mary just kept struggling. Other members on board crowded around the stern, shouting encouragement: "Come on, Mary. Don't give up. Drop the rock!"

Their encouragement gave Mary a boost of energy, but she realized that every new effort forward met resistance from something heavy around her neck, which she was just now becoming aware of. She didn't know what it was, and so she just tried harder, making a little progress before running out of breath again.

She looked up and saw all her friends on the boat, holding out their hands and hollering for her to keep swimming. But the heavy weight was winning, and she understood in a flash that she would go down for the third and last time if she didn't get rid of what was pulling her under.

This thing around her neck—it was something she had brought with her, Mary now realized. That's what they were all trying to tell her—to let go of what she had been carrying that was taking her down just when she was within sight of rescue—resentments, fear, dishonesty, self-pity, intolerance, anger. Those were just some of the things that formed her rock.

God, help me get rid of this rock, she prayed. *Please—now!*

Kicking desperately to stay afloat, she began yanking off the strings holding the boulder around her neck and felt her load begin to lighten. With one more burst of energy, she was able to let go of her burden. Amazed at how easy the swimming had become, she caught up with the boat, and her friends hauled her up out of the water onto the safety of the deck.

This group milled around, congratulating Mary for her accomplishment, praising her, and declaring how much fun they were all going to have together as they headed out to the island. The scare behind her, Mary dried off with gratitude and relief. As she was thinking how good it was going to feel to rest and relax, she looked back at where she had just come from. Something near the pier caught her attention.

Something—or rather, some*one*—was bobbing in the water. "Look!" she cried out to the group, seeing their smiles replaced by concern as she pointed to what looked like a person going under the water. She was first to the stern, leaning over and shouting, "Hey, friend, drop the rock!"[1]

I have never been a great swimmer. Indeed, my high school swim teacher Mr. Bluck christened me "Broken Buoy" because I couldn't perform a dead man's float without sinking. I gave Mr. Bluck a nickname too. It rhymed with his last name. I screamed it at him whenever I was at the bottom of the pool.

I need not elaborate.

As a young adult, however, I learned how to swim fairly well in the "ocean of myself." Most of us do. It's the way of things. As we mature, we gradually learn about our inner workings and unconsciously devise ways to protect our hearts from the assaults that life regularly launches against us. Over time and with practice, we begin to assume that we really know ourselves.

But in every life, there come moments when we realize we don't know ourselves nearly as well as we think we do. We find ourselves acting, thinking, and feeling in ways that shock us. Waves heave and swell, and we feel the weight of our flaws and shortcomings dragging us under. Like Mary, we must find a way to "drop the rock" of our character defects or drown, which is what Steps Six and Seven are designed to help us do.

In treatment, I saw how my many self-defeating behaviors prevented me from making progress on my spiritual journey. Embarrassingly, my character defects show up in my life with such regularity and predictability that I can set my watch to them. The fallout that results from my occasional buffoonery isn't always serious. Talking too much, chewing loudly, or not always being punctual makes one annoying—not a hopeless moral reprobate. That said, I have other "character defects" that cause me and others to suffer in ways that break my heart. I trust you can relate. But don't despair! I'm about to throw us a life ring.

I was emotionally and spiritually exhausted after finishing my Fourth and Fifth Steps. So I was ecstatic when I read Steps Six and Seven for the first time. "Compared to working Steps Four and Five, these Steps will be a cinch," I told Sponsor Steve when we first met to begin work on Steps Six and Seven. "Honestly, who doesn't want God to remove all their character defects?"

It was a record-scratch moment when Sponsor Steve told me that Steps Six and Seven are arguably the most difficult of the Twelve Steps. Bill Wilson quotes a friend of A.A. as saying that Step Six is the Step that "separates the men [women] from the boys [girls]."[2] I would say the same applies to Step Seven.

It's a common misconception that Steps Six and Seven are easily and quickly completed. Thus people working the Steps for the first time tend to downplay their importance and zip through them, which explains why they're called "the Flyover Steps" or "the Forgotten Steps." It's understandable when you think about it. When you read these two Steps, it almost looks like all we have to do is sit on our butts, become "ready for God" to remove our character defects, and then humbly ask him to do so. It all sounds so breezy and effortless that nobody could fault you for thinking you could blow through these two Steps while lounging in a deck chair on a yacht lazily cruising the Mediterranean. Well, abandon ship, kids. Steps Six and

Seven sound straightforward and undemanding, but they're anything but. This is where you become ready and willing to let God transform you at the molecular level. This is the very heart of the program.

There's a brilliant inner logic to the Steps. They stack and build perfectly on each other. In Step One, we admitted our powerlessness over our addictions or recurrent addictive behaviors (not to mention over pretty much everything else in life). In Step Two, we came to believe that someone or something could save us, and in Step Three, we turned our will and lives over to the care of God as we understood him. So far, so good, right? Then in Step Four, we reviewed our histories and rummaged around in our shadows to uncover our defects of character—our resentments, selfishness, self-centeredness, self-pity, our debilitating fears, and the many other "manifestations of self" that have alienated us not only from our higher power but also from ourselves and others. In Step Five, we admitted our defects of character and wrongdoings to God, ourselves, and another human being.

Now, when we arrive at Steps Six and Seven, we realize that the Twelve Steps aren't merely about overcoming our addictions. They're a total life makeover! Again, we come to understand that our addictions weren't the problem; they were a *symptom* of our problem—namely, our feeling of not-at-homeness, the escape we wanted from the pain of our unresolved traumas, our wanting to play God and control *everything* in life (others, circumstances, outcomes). The Steps reveal the errant patterns of thinking, feeling, and behaving that drive our addictions, and they offer us a lifelong design for living in a spiritually and emotionally sober manner.

In Steps Six and Seven, we become ready to have God relieve us of the burden of these shortcomings. It's time to hand over all your character defects—obstacles to your spiritually waking up and gaining a new relationship with God—to God that were revealed in Steps Four and Five. Trust me, if you choose to follow the Twelve-Step path, you will work Steps Six and Seven daily for the rest of your life.

If here at the halfway point on our journey through the Steps we face and successfully surrender our character defects to God, we will undergo a psychic change and spiritual transformation at a depth we've likely never experienced.

Before we go any further, let me define what I mean when I use the term *character defects*. A character defect is any behavior that blocks the love of God from flowing in us and through us into the world. It is any pattern of behavior that stands in the way of our usefulness to God and others. These misguided, mostly fear-based behaviors undermine our relationships and underwrite our addictions.

Personally, I don't like to think of my flaws or sins *only* as "character defects." I have enough shame in my life. I don't need to heap more on myself by labeling myself "defective." I prefer the term *character defenses* because I can't think of a single wrongdoing or sin I've ever committed that wasn't a disorganized and misguided attempt to meet a basic human need that went unmet in childhood. Most of my character defects began as defensive strategies that helped me survive and care for myself in childhood in a way I thought none of my caretakers would.

For example, as a kid, my parents were too consumed with their own problems to acknowledge my gifts and accomplishments. Thus, I became starved for love and attention. So, what's a little tyke to do? My clever mind unconsciously thought, *What if I talk up my wins and maybe even embellish them a little in the hope that someone will see and praise me?*

On one level, this plan worked. A few friends, teachers, and coaches patted me on the head for my achievements. In time, however, I developed what I now call my "attaboy!" addiction. It's embarrassing, but there are still days when my long-standing need for approval born of childhood neglect pops up again like a carnival whack-a-mole. If I don't watch myself, I'll drop the name of a well-known friend or humbly brag about a flattering book review or "big deal" speaking invitation in a bid to win the approval and love of others.

In childhood, I also learned to occasionally lie or "landscape the truth" to avoid harsh punishments that were frequently disproportionate to the crime. Devoid of guidance from my parents, I also developed an "inner parent" who would harshly punish me for even my smallest mistakes to ensure I wouldn't make them again. This led to a soul-crushing perfectionism that periodically still prosecutes me for making even the most basic of human errors. I also discovered I could prop up my wobbly self-esteem and make myself feel superior to others if I subtly (or not-so-subtly) put people down behind their backs.

Approval addiction, name-dropping, lying, perfectionism, and the occasional trash talk—all of these and my other character defenses developed to help me feel in control, soothe my pain, and get my needs met in a chaotic and unpredictable world. I adopted these nutty strategies long before I knew about a higher power who could tell me I was beloved, who could provide for me. I unconsciously brought these character defenses into adulthood, where they regularly make a mess of things. Lord, have mercy!

This is why working a Twelve-Step program with *a lot* of self-compassion is so important. It's usually our conscious and unconscious fears that activate our character defenses. (Hence, the importance of doing a fear inventory!) To overcome them, we must be honest and gentle with ourselves. Take it from me—you can't hate yourself into becoming a more loving person. I've tried. Obsessing about your imperfect nature and beating yourself up for having character defects is itself a character defect. Be kind—we do what we do in life to survive. The good news? We can heal and change.

Challenges

Working Step Six presents us with a number of challenges I need to give you a heads-up about so you can head them off at the pass.

Your Sly Ego

All of us want to be free of our self-defeating behaviors (at least a few of them), but our ego will sneakily try to take charge of the process. It wants us to believe that Step Six reads, "Became entirely ready to make my character defects [defenses] go away *by virtue of sheer willpower.*" Good luck with that, y'all.

And here's a sly move: your ego will smile and give God credit for any small "success" you might have with overcoming your character defects on your own. This is a cringey form of spiritual pride. Keep your eye on that ego. She's an impish creature.

Instincts Run Riot

In *Twelve Steps and Twelve Traditions*, Bill Wilson writes, "The chief activator of our defects has been self-centered fear—primarily fear that we would lose something we already possessed or would fail to get something we demanded. Living upon a basis of unsatisfied demands, we were in a state of continual disturbance and frustration. Therefore, no peace was to be had unless we could find a means of reducing these demands. The difference between a demand and a simple request is plain to anyone."[3]

All humans have powerful, God-given instincts that help keep them alive. At the very least, they include security and safety, esteem and approval, love and sex, and a need for mastery and reasonable control. It's impossible to overstate how much power these basic needs and instincts exercise over our thoughts, feelings, actions, and decisions. Disaster awaits when the demands of our basic human instincts swell and become overblown and collide with the outsized instincts of other people.

There's eventually going to be a whole heap of trouble at the office if our need for approval and security swells and inspires us to speak ill of a colleague to make ourselves look good. If our instinct for romance overinflates and we become clingy and codependent with another person, we will eventually smother them and be rejected. If we fear that we're losing control over our lives and we manipulate or bully to feel more secure, people will strike back at us.

These are but a few of the ways our overblown instincts create fear, which triggers character defects, which causes misery, which arouses our need for soothing and addiction. Oh dear, here we are again.

We need to be aware of the terrible power of our swollen instincts while we work on Step Six. These instincts might try to convince us that we can't give up the character defects that are designed to protect and satisfy them.

Timing

While in treatment, I composed a list of character defects or defenses that I was committed to working on when I returned home. The first one on my list was conflict avoidance. Seriously, I prayed about it. I journaled about it. I put sticky notes on my bathroom mirror and on the dashboard of my car that read, "Pull up your socks, man!" But my fear of conflict wouldn't budge. However, while I was laboring to dismantle that defense, my lifelong fear of economic insecurity mysteriously evaporated without any effort on my part. Apparently, God gets to pick which of my character defenses he wants to work on first.

No Hacks

People are always looking for hacks to cut down on the amount of time and effort it takes to mature in the spiritual life. They buy books that outline simple steps and promise an "easier and softer way" for quicker results. Every great spiritual master would laugh at us for believing this nonsense. Listen, it's impossible to hack the spiritual life. *Repeat*—there are no techniques, plans, or workarounds that will lead to

union with God *overnight*. I know of few programs that produce the kind of radical change the Twelve Steps do, but even
the early pioneers of the recovery movement admitted that
deep transformation takes time, and that's okay. "Sometimes
quickly, sometimes slowly," Bill Wilson wrote.[4] Abandon the
idea that you will become "sober Jesus" anytime soon.

Fear of Change

I'm from the Northeast. I could teach sarcasm as a second
language. Honestly, I enjoy dark humor, the verbal jab and
parry, the competition to land the cleverest dig. Sorry, it's my
love language. I'm only half as snarky as I used to be, but I
have a ways to go. While working my Sixth Step, I examined
my "communication style" and became aware my speech was
often too harsh, not to mention the fact that it's an unconscious
strategy to keep people from getting too close to me. Working
through the Steps, I realized that my teasing banter sometimes
made me an unsafe person.

If I'm completely honest, I'd say part of me wanted God
to remove this shortcoming and part of me was terrified he
would. Like all human beings, I was afraid of change. I had
overidentified who I was with "being a wise guy." People had
come to expect it of me. Some folks even thought it was funny.
"Who will I be if I'm not at least a little Larry David-ish?"
I half-joked with my fellow recovery pal Casey.

"Don't worry, you'll be the same jerk you were before," he
said, putting his arm around my shoulder. Casey is from the
Northeast too. I should have asked someone from Iowa.

It's frightening to confront and dismantle character
defenses you've employed since childhood to get your needs

met. We don't get to bargain either. We can't say to God, "Let's make a deal. I'll hand over 75 percent of my lust if you let me retain a 25 percent minority share. We good?" Like it or not, the program says we must be willing to go to any length to achieve recovery—all or nothing. That means we need to be *entirely ready* to have God remove *all* our shortcomings, not only a few or a percentage thereof. If we find ourselves bargaining with God, our ego is back at the wheel.

Impatience

No one likes to wait, but it's how the world works. If you'd like to practice patience, purposely go to the DMV, fill out the wrong forms, wait in line for three hours, and be told to go to the back of the queue. Or you could take the words of the great Pierre Teilhard de Chardin to heart: "Above all, trust in the slow work of God,"[5] and get on with your day.

Most of our character defenses will not instantly disappear (though some might!). Many are deeply grooved into our neural pathways, and God may take his time dealing with them, even when we'd like him to get on with it. Look at your list of character defenses twenty years from now, and you'll find some that are still on it. We're not in charge of anything. God decides which character defenses he will remove, when he will remove them, and how he will remove them. Trust him to do the work.

How to Work the Sixth and Seventh Steps

You may tire of hearing me say this, but the gospel and the Twelve Steps are about powerlessness, willingness, acceptance, honesty, open-mindedness, and surrender. *We don't do the steps; God does.* Our part in the bargain is to pray for the alacrity to let God do the work in us. Or as my friend Graham likes to say, "We supply the willingness, and God supplies the change."

That said, we can help create the natural climate in which we can open ourselves to the work of grace and change. Here are a few practices I've used to cooperate with God's grace.

Pray for the Gift of Humility

Several years ago, my wife, Anne, asked me to go to her hot yoga class, where I quickly learned the difference between humility and humiliation.

I'd never been to a hot yoga class, but she was tired of hearing me dismiss it as a workout for people who had aged out of doing "real exercise." I should have known better. Anne might qualify for AARP discounts, but she still has a six-pack. I kid you not, you could drop a quarter on her abs and it would bounce back and take out your eye. This woman would not waste her time doing an easy workout.

I was the only man in the class that day, and when I walked into the studio, I thought, *Dang, it's roasting in here.* That's because hot yoga takes place in a studio that's cooked to 105 degrees with 40 percent humidity. Still, I thought, *I'll show these Lulu girls how this is done.*

I wasn't ten minutes into class however before I discovered that hot yoga is what you do when you want to give yourself a spinal injury and an excuse for taking several months off from work. It was while practicing a yoga posture called the Eagle Pose that things went sideways. Eagle involves bending your knees, crossing your right thigh over your left, then hooking the top of your foot behind your left calf. At the same time, you have to snug your left elbow into the crook of your right and stretch your fingers toward the ceiling.

"Wring yourself out like a dish towel," the instructor yelled at us. Refusing to admit defeat, I squeezed until the unthinkable happened.

I farted.

Friends, I'm not talking about a polite *poof*. No. This was a full-throated gaseous proclamation of my attendance in the class. A moment of silence that felt like an eternity passed before Anne snorted, which led to the entire class falling out of Eagle Pose and laughing. Though it was brief, what I felt in that moment was humiliation, the feeling that I was "naked and ashamed." Humiliation involves being brought low, a loss of pride and self-respect.

But toward the end of the class I learned about humility. When I was on the precipice of heat stroke, the instructor said, "Give yourself permission to lie down on your mat if you're feeling overwhelmed. Lying down requires humility, which is why we say it's the most difficult of all the postures."

Humility is starkly different from humiliation. Humility is having a clear-eyed estimation of who you are and who you aren't. It's knowing your limitations, what's best about you, and what needs work. A person who is humble neither overvalues nor undervalues themselves. They know they're no better or worse than anyone else. They don't need to sit in the front or the back of the boat. They're happy to sit in the middle with everyone else.

More than anything else, you will need humility to complete Steps Six and Seven. You must admit you're at the end of your rope and lie down. If it sounds terrible, it's not.

Thomas Merton wrote, "In humility is the greatest freedom,"[6] because it is only in humility that we accept the truth about ourselves and find hope for our restoration.

Make a List

I reviewed and wrote down all the character defenses I could first identify while working on my Fourth and Fifth steps. Once I finished, Sponsor Steve gave me a list of character defenses I hadn't considered, kind man that he is. I've included that list in the workbook so you can reflect on it as well.

For me, the Enneagram proved to be one of several resources that helped bring into conscious awareness the character defenses I'd been blind to. If you're familiar with the Enneagram, you know each of the nine types contends with their own shortcomings and deadly sins. Of course, there's bleedover. For example, I'm an Enneagram Four, but I occasionally battle with perfectionism like Ones do.

Read your type below, and notice a few of its hallmark defects and defenses. While these are only a handful, reviewing these summaries can provide a useful starting place for putting together your list of shortcomings. I've included a more exhaustive list in the workbook.

> **Enneagram Ones**—Resentment, fear of change, perfectionism, closed-mindedness, dualistic thinking, impatience, intolerance, judgmentalism, being critical, rigidity, defensiveness, deflecting blame, needing to be right, self-righteousness, an unforgiving spirit, overactive inner critic, belief that their way is the only correct way, preachy.

Enneagram Twos—Pride, codependency, overly focused on the needs of others, disavowing their own feelings and needs, believing they know the needs of others better than they actually do, controlling behavior, manipulation, resentment, expects others to know and meet their needs without having to acknowledge them, pretending to like people they don't, self-pity.

Enneagram Threes—Image management, narcissistic behavior, focusing more on externals than internals, overvaluing success and the admiration of others, chameleon-like behavior, cutting corners to ensure success, workaholism, accumulating status symbols, self-marketing, self-deceit, insincerity, performing feelings rather than having feelings, embellishing achievements, boastful, too socially and professionally competitive, vanity.

Enneagram Fours—Self-absorption, overidentifying with feelings, envy, jealousy, perfectionism, focusing on an idealized past and future, fixing attention on what's missing, taking things personally, ingratitude, unstable relationships, elitism, dependency, believing they're special and unique, fantasizing, self-pity, superior, ungrateful, comparing self to others.

Enneagram Fives—Avarice, hoarding time and material resources, privacy and personal autonomy, emotional unavailability, intellectual snobbery, aloof, overfocus on self-sufficiency and independence, miserliness.

Enneagram Sixes—Fear, future tripping, dependency on authority figures, indecisiveness, pessimism, paranoia, suspicious, distrusting, anxious, worried.

Enneagram Sevens—Lack of empathy, gluttony for interesting experiences and stimulation, fear of suffering and painful feelings, difficulty remaining in the present moment, tendency toward addictive behavior, dishonesty, reframing, rationalizing questionable behaviors and decisions, self-justification, impulsive, self-important, thrill-seeking, promise-breaking.

Enneagram Eights—Controlling others and the environment to mask vulnerability, combativeness, domineering, intimidation, impulsive decision-making, overly autocratic, making rules for others while breaking them, difficulty apologizing, dismissing those who aren't as strong as they are, oppositional, obstructive, sarcastic, excessive.

Enneagram Nines—Sloth, laziness, merging with the agenda of groups and individuals, self-abandonment and self-negation, distractibility, dependency, codependency, passive-aggressive anger, stubbornness, dishonesty when stressed, apathetic, failure to self-invest, conflict avoidant, forgetful, lack of purpose, procrastination, denying anger, resisting growth.

Character Defense Jar

On the kitchen counter in my home, I have a large Mason jar that contains small slips of paper on which are written my many character defects. Every morning, I pull one of those slips out and set an intention. Let's say I pull the slip out that reads "procrastination." I first ask myself if I'm *really* willing to let God remove that character defect. If I'm not, I pray, *God, help me at least to become willing to become willing to let this behavior go.*

But if I am ready to let procrastination go, I (hopefully) humbly ask God to take procrastination from me. From time to time, God instantly removes a character defect from someone, but these "Our Lady of Lourdes-like" exorcisms are pretty darn rare. So I put that slip of paper in my pocket to remind me to practice diligence that day—the opposite of procrastination. Ignatius of Loyola called this exercise *agere contra*, which means "acting against" your normal pattern to interrupt the circuit of your habitual self-defeating behavior patterns.

Though it might not immediately eliminate procrastination from my life, using my Sixth Step jar has weakened its death grip on my life.

Rationalization

If we're honest, we'll admit we actually enjoy many of our character defenses. For some folks, sloth is yummy. For others, self-righteous indignation is scrumptious. I don't know which personal shortcomings you don't want to let go of, but "everybody got something." And so, in a bid to protect and preserve our favorite character defenses, we make excuses for them. We tell ourselves they're only petty offenses. If we're particularly self-deceived, we paint our character defenses as virtues. For example, we might reveal confidential information about an acquaintance with another person (that's called gossip) and tell them we're sharing it because the poor soul "needs our prayers" (that's called a twisted self-justification). Beware of rationalization!

Prayer

If there's one spiritual discipline the Twelve Steps encourage, it's prayer. The first thing I do every morning when I get up is get on my knees and pray the "Seventh Step Prayer" found in *The Big Book*: "My Creator, I am now willing that you should have all of me, good and bad. I pray that you now remove from me every single defect of character which stands in the way of my usefulness to you and my fellows. Grant me strength, as I go out from here, to do your bidding."[7]

That's about as good a way to start the day as any, don't you think?

Meditation and Centering Prayer

Mindfulness meditation and centering prayer are two of the most essential and effective practices I know for sharpening the attentional muscle in our brain that can spot and alert us when our ego and character defenses have been activated and taken over. I'll talk more about these practices when we get to Step Eleven!

Journaling

I used to hate journaling. Seriously, I loathed it. Whenever I read one of those spiritual formation books that claimed journaling was an essential discipline for Christian spiritual growth, I wanted to become a Scientologist.

Then I did the research.

Researchers from the University of Texas at Austin, among other institutions, have shown that regular journaling helps people make sense of trauma, understand their emotions, improve their mood, overcome anxiety and depression, and strengthen their immune system.[8] Who knew journaling could help me ward off the flu?

Journaling about my character defects has aided me in countless ways. It has helped me dispassionately identify and compassionately work through my shortcomings.

"Me Too" Friendships

My best friends Pete and Michael are in recovery. On Sunday nights, we have our own little Twelve-Step meeting during which we share where we are on our recovery journey. We don't mess around. We openly discuss things about ourselves that we wouldn't tell anyone else in a million years, and we do it because we know that addictions, like mold, grow like crazy in the dark. We all need a few trusted friends with whom we can share the ongoing battle we're having with our character defects so we can hear another person say, "Me too." Shame hates those words.

Rituals

We underestimate the power of rituals to mark transitions and intentions. Recently, a friend named Stuart, who was in early recovery from a sex addiction, gathered a few of us together for cigars around the firepit behind his farm. Sitting around the fire, he told us about how he now avoided going into his home office because it's where he would sit on his couch and watch porn. It was too triggering and painful to return to the scene of the crime.

"Let's torch the couch," our friend Graham said.

"What?" Stuart said incredulously.

"Let's do it!" we all chimed in, running into the house to grab it.

That night, a group of six broken brothers played the Beatles song *Let It Be* on an iPhone and "cooked the sofa," as we now refer to it. Weird as it was, it turned out to be a powerful, laughter-and-tear-filled way to mark Stuart's rebirth. None of us will ever forget it.

When my friend Teresa, who is in OA for an eating addiction, finished her Sixth Step, she threw a party for her character defenses to thank them for helping her survive in childhood and to let them know she didn't need them anymore. What a celebration that was!

All to say, tap into the magic of rituals to mark the completion of your Sixth and Seventh Steps.

Let Go and Let God

"Do you want to be healed?" (John 5:6 RSV). This question posed by Jesus to the man by the pool at Bethsaida moves me. God is respectful of the freedom he has given us. He won't remove our character defenses without our permission. Therefore, I suggest you daily attempt to adopt the posture of Mary, who, when told she would give birth to the Messiah, said, "Let it be done to me according to your word" (Luke 1:38 NCB), not "Cool, I'll take it from here."

You will repeatedly work Steps Six and Seven throughout your recovery journey. Again, don't be discouraged if you see defects on your list twenty years from now—ones that God hasn't removed yet. The Twelve Steps aren't a competition against yourself. As Bill Wilson wrote, "No one among us has been able to maintain anything like perfect adherence to these principles. We are not saints. The point is, that we are willing to grow along spiritual lines. The principles we have set down are guides to progress. We claim spiritual progress rather than spiritual perfection."[9]

Or as my Mexican priest friend Ronaldo says every time we take leave of each other, *"Todo es gracia."* All is grace.

I'm banking on it.

Chapter Nine

MEA CULPA

**We're all just waiting for our
moment to redeem ourselves.**
Philip Elliott, *Hunger and Hallelujahs*

STEP EIGHT

**Made a list of all persons we had harmed,
and became willing to make amends to them all.**

STEP NINE

**Made direct amends to such people wherever possible,
except when to do so would injure them or others.**

The legendary Dr. Seuss summarizes the message of the
Eighth and Ninth Steps in his wonderful story *Bartholomew
and the Oobleck* in which Dr. Seuss invites kids to question
authority figures who abuse their power.

In it, an overindulged king is bored by the weather and
orders his page Bartholomew Cubbins to summon the royal
magicians to pull out of the sky something more interesting
than the usual sunshine, rain, fog, and snow.

At first, the king is overjoyed by their creation of
oobleck—a sticky green substance that fell from the sky—but
it soon floods and gums up the entire kingdom, including
the palace. Panicked, the king orders Bartholomew (who had
thought the whole plan was a dumb idea from the start) to
instruct the magicians to reverse their magic. But Bartholomew
tells the king that the magicians are helplessly mired in goo,
just like everyone else in the kingdom. They are trapped inside

their mountain lab and unable to act. Then Bartholomew dares suggest that the king man up and simply apologize for his stupidity.

At first, the king is indignant that his lowly page would challenge his authority. But when Bartholomew presses his point and declares him no sort of a king at all if he can't take responsibility for the havoc his choice has wreaked, the king finally breaks down and sobs out an apology.

The moment the king utters, "You're right! It *is* all my fault! And I *am* sorry! . . . I'm awfully, *awfully* sorry," the sun comes out, the oobleck melts away, and the world returns to normal. The king praises his young page's heroism, and all's well that ends well.

What's the lesson? In the words of Dr. Seuss, "Maybe there *was* something magic in those simple words 'I'm sorry. Maybe there *was* something magic in those simple words, 'It's all my fault.'"[1] When a plea for forgiveness is expressed sincerely, it can change everything. But when the words remain unspoken, they can embitter and imprison a person for life.

I've never met anyone who doesn't ache to hear an acknowledgment of wrongdoing and the words "please forgive me" from someone who hurt them in their past. In my first year of practice as a psychotherapist, I met weekly with an eighty-five-year-old client named Terence, whose mother had packed up and deserted him and his father in the middle of the night when he was ten years old. "If only I could have heard her say she was sorry," he once said to me through tears. "Maybe my life would have turned out differently." Terence was right. If his mother had expressed remorse and made amends for abandoning her family, perhaps he wouldn't have spent seventy-five years believing her departure was his fault.

And what about you? How would your life be different if someone who once wounded or betrayed you finally owned up to their mistakes and asked how they could make it up to you? It would change things for you, right? Maybe *a lot* of things.

So in Step Eight, the program asks us to face an uncomfortable truth—none of us get off this troubled earth without hurting at least a few—and, in some cases, a lot of—people. To advance the cause of shalom, the ancient Hebrew concept of peace and ultimate well-being, we must take responsibility for *our* actions and make amends to those *we* have harmed. As part of this movement toward repairing ruptured relationships, we will have to forgive ourselves and others as well.

If you think this journey through the Twelve Steps is beginning to feel like a scene from the cheerless film *Manchester by the Sea*, take a breath and remind yourself that if you complete this Step, your life (and the lives of a few other people you know) is about to get a whole lot happier. Spiritually speaking, Steps Eight and Nine are juicy fare. When you get done with them, you will be released from the burden of shame, fear, sadness, regret, guilt, and resentment that dog you. This is the beginning of the end of your feeling of being alienated from God, yourself, and others. Soon you will be free. You have a lot to look forward to!

Because you're an intelligent person, I'm sure you are seeing a pattern emerge. Steps One through Three concern themselves with healing your relationship with *God*, Steps Four through Seven focus on mending your relationship with *yourself*, and now, Steps Eight and Nine are about repairing your relationship with *others*. This is a formula for happiness and serenity. In Steps Eight and Nine, you will receive instructions on how to clean up any relational wreckage you might have in your past, as well as how to make things right with those you have hurt along life's way.

There are two parts to Step Eight: first we're asked to make a list of all the people we have harmed, the second part asks us to "become willing" to make amends to them all.

Challenges

Make a list. Sounds simple, right? It's more difficult than it sounds.

From the get-go, that puckish ego of yours will duck and dive to avoid taking this humbling and scary step. The last thing it wants to do is admit fault or blame. Be forewarned— your ego has lots of tricks up its sleeve.

The first is procrastination. *What exactly constitutes a harm?* your ego might ask, gazing detachedly into the distance, nibbling the eraser at the end of her pencil. Of course, this is goldbricking. You don't need to consult an expert in moral philosophy to define the term *harm*. If you're not sure what qualifies as harm, simply write down anything anyone has ever done or said to you that made you feel angry, resentful, hurt, ashamed, sad, or afraid, and then put to paper the names of all the people *you* have hurt by doing those very same things to *them*. That should give you plenty of petrol to prime the list-writing pump.

To skirt having to own up to hurting other people, your ego might also choose to *explain* a hurtful episode rather than admit wrongdoing and make amends for it. *I'm sorry, but I had just found out that Starbucks might discontinue making pumpkin spice lattes when I punched you in the face.* (Oh, that's alright then.)

Or your ego might allow you to make a list of people it can't deny harming but then immediately rush to its own defense by proposing a comparison to justify its misdeeds. *Sure, I poured coffee on his computer,* the ego protests, *but he took credit for my work with the boss. Isn't that worse?* But Step Eight isn't concerned with what the other person did or didn't do to you. This is about *you* owning *your* part and sweeping *your* side of the street. This is not your chance to present the other person's crime sheet to the prosecutor, only yours.

Finally, a common self-sabotaging mistake people make when working on Steps Eight and Nine is conflating them. All you are asked to do in Step Eight is make a list of people you've hurt and become *willing* to make things right with them. *And that's it. Nada más.*

That is to say, don't start making movies in your head filled with scenes of how intolerably awkward your face-to-face amends conversations will be with your judgy sister-in-law. If you start future-tripping about making amends at this early stage, you will panic and be tempted to put off taking this Step altogether. We'll talk about what might or might not happen when you actually begin having amends conversations with people in Step Nine. Don't worry, you'll be alright. For now, just make the list!

The best way to start your list is with prayer. Simply ask God to bring to your mind the names of everyone you have

ever physically, emotionally, mentally, spiritually, professionally, sexually, or financially harmed in your life. That's right,
Step Eight says to write down the names of *all* the people you
have ever hurt, so it doesn't matter how small the misdeed or
how long ago it occurred—just write it down.

I began populating my amends list with the names of
all the people closest to me (friends and family) whom I had
ever hurt, before, during, or after I was in my active addiction. Then I added the people on my Fourth Step Resentment
and Sexual Conduct Inventory lists. To further jog my woolly
memory, I then scrolled through all eleven hundred people in
my iPhone's contact list, paged through old high school and
college yearbooks, and asked my closest friends if they knew
of anyone to whom I needed to make amends.

Now, don't come unglued if your list is long. When you're
finished, you and your sponsor (hopefully you have one by
now!) will comb through it and "cull the herd"—removing
from it the names of people who probably don't need to be on
it. For example, your second-grade classmate Howie probably
doesn't need you to apologize and Venmo him the lunch
money you swiped from him in 1998. I think Howie's over it
by now, don't you? That said, it's important to acknowledge
to yourself and God that you once hurt Howie. There's healing power in that admission. Now let it go. You have bigger
fish to fry.

Next to the name of every person on your now pared-
down amends list write down:

- their contact information
- a brief description of how you harmed them

- thoughts about why you did what you did, and how you feel about it now
- the specific amends you think will restore balance to the relationship

Now, don't be surprised if while reading over your list, it surfaces painful stuff for you. I would be worried about the state of your soul if it didn't. As hard as it may be, you have to grieve your wrongs. You need to feel what the other person felt when you hurt them, or you won't change. Your addictions are, in part, strategies for numbing those old feelings, so you have to experience them to render the addiction unnecessary. Again, please note, this Step doesn't say, "Made a list of all people we had harmed and became willing to eternally torture ourselves for being horrid wretches." Be kind, people, be kind.

Amends, Apologies, and Forgiveness

To be clear, an amends differs from an apology. An apology is when we merely say "I'm sorry" to someone we've hurt. Now, don't get me wrong, simple apologies make sense for the little stuff (e.g., running over someone's foot with your shopping cart), but not when you really hurt someone (e.g., abandoning a friend in their hour of need). The word *apology* derives from the Latin *apologia*, which means "to speak in defense of an action," which is precisely what no one wants to hear us do when we've seriously wronged them.

If we're honest, we will admit that merely saying "I'm sorry" is often a manipulative dodge. It's a way to pacify the person we've harmed and get them to say that "everything's cool" so we can move on without having to change our behavior or "feel all the bad feels" for our acting like half-wits. Furthermore, saying "I'm sorry" often leaves the apologizer in charge. At times, an apology has a "There I said it; now let's move on" quality to it. Uh-uh, that won't do.

Another reason saying "I'm sorry" isn't sufficient is because we've likely said it so many times that it means very little to people now. "I'm sorry I lied again about watching porn." "I'm sorry I'm a workaholic who sneaks off to take work calls on family vacations when I promised I wouldn't do that anymore." "I'm sorry I keep compulsively sneaking food, being overly critical, or passively-aggressively controlling everyone."

When making your amends, I encourage you to specifically ask for forgiveness rather than merely say "I'm sorry." This is not simply a matter of semantics. When an offender says, "Will you please forgive me?" they make themselves vulnerable by giving the harmed person the power and dignity to choose whether to accept the request or not. Saying "I ask your forgiveness" has an "I place myself at your mercy" quality to it. It's more complete and full.

Now that you know what an amends isn't, let's talk about what it is. When you make amends, you not only ask forgiveness, but you also take concrete steps to make things right with the person you've hurt. For instance, imagine you key your friend Crystal's car because you mistakenly thought she was flirting with your boyfriend. Would merely pleading temporary insanity and saying you're sorry to Crystal for carving your initials into the hood of her Camry be enough to restore balance to your relationship with her? I think not. To make things right, you should not only ask Crystal for forgiveness (that's important), *but* also offer to make amends by paying to get a new paint job for her car as well. Crystal would then know you're serious about repairing the rupture you caused in your relationship with her. (By the way, you should give Crystal a gift certificate to a nail salon for a year's worth of pedicures as well. You keyed her dang car!)

Making amends is what the tax collector Zacchaeus from Bible days did when he was confronted with his sin of stealing money from people, and his contrite heart got Jesus' attention:

> But Zacchaeus stood up and said to the Lord, "Look, Lord! Here and now I give half of my possessions to the poor, and if I have cheated anybody out of anything, I will pay back four times the amount."
>
> Jesus said to him, "Today salvation has come to this house, because this man, too, is a son of Abraham. For the Son of Man came to seek and to save the lost." (Luke 19:8–10)

Became Willing

When I completed my list, I was *willing* to make things right with almost all the people on it. I knew the conversations I would have with some of them would be uncomfortable, but I was still prepared to have them.

But then there were "those people." *Those* people fell under the rubric of "Heck, no! I'm never making amends to that schmuck." The people on my "schmuck list" were folks who in my estimation had harmed me far more egregiously than I had harmed them in the past, and in many cases my conclusion was true. I could not get my head around the idea that I needed to go to those people to acknowledge my part in the breakdown of our relationship *and* make amends to *them* for it.

Was I willing? Heck, no, pal. It's hard to admit, but spiritually speaking, this felt way too advanced for me. I've asked for forgiveness and made things right with lots of people, but there are still folks on my schmuck list with whom I'm still not willing to make amends because I'm still working on forgiving them. Not to put too fine a point on it, but I would rather eat broken glass and die than put my tail between my legs and make amends with a few of the people on my schmuck list.

Bill Wilson was a brilliant student of human nature. He didn't presume that once we completed our list, we would immediately be willing to make amends to everyone on it. In fact, it's often a bad idea to try to make amends to someone you haven't first forgiven for hurting you. He knew we would have to forgive the people on our schmuck list before we could go to them to make a *sincere* amends. If you go to one of these people without first forgiving them for what they did to you, your amends will probably ring hollow, or you will leak contempt, make an indirectly hostile jab, or mention their mistakes and end up in a verbal brawl. Now listen, forgiving your schmucks doesn't mean they win. Trust me, *you* do. But it can take a minute.

I have a person on my amends list who hurt me terribly. Yes, I played a role in the flameout of our friendship, but I don't believe I did nearly as many harmful things to them as they did to me. But here's what I did: I told God I would take the hint and make my amends if he arranged it so that I would run into this person somewhere at some point (e.g., at a speaking event, at a restaurant, or in a hotel restroom). I then secretly hoped that encounter would never happen. (Just being honest.) That said, I've made it a point to "never say never" and I regularly pray, *Lord, help me at least be willing to be willing to forgive and make amends to this person.* As Bill Wilson counseled, "If we haven't the will to do this, we ask until it comes."[2]

Now, I know what you're thinking: *This sounds great in theory, but how do I forgive someone who really hurt me?* Well, let me offer a prayer practice I promise can help you let go of old resentments and open your heart to forgiving those who harmed you, even those who deeply hurt you.

First, sit comfortably, close your eyes, and take a few deep cleansing breaths. Ask the Spirit of God to surround you. When you're feeling grounded, bring your attention to the area around your heart, imagining a picture of yourself in your mind's eye. I find that if I place my hand on my heart, it helps me connect to the experience. For two minutes, direct words of loving-kindness toward yourself by slowly repeating these phrases, which are timed with your inhalations and exhalations.

May I have love (inhale).
May I have joy (exhale).
May I have peace (inhale).
May I have healing (exhale).
May I have rest (inhale).

After two minutes have expired, transition to picturing someone in your mind whom you deeply love. This could be a friend, your partner, one of your kids, a pet, or anyone who arouses in you immediate feelings of warmth and affection. Now direct the same phrases of loving-kindness and good intention toward this person for two minutes. *If your mind wanders (and it will!) gently return your attention to your breath and the suggested phrases.*

May you have love (inhale).
May you have joy (exhale).
May you have peace (inhale).
May you have healing (exhale).
May you have rest (inhale).

That feels good, right? Well, here comes the challenging bit. Bring to mind a mental picture of the person who harmed you—the person you have long struggled to forgive. Allow your heart to open and gentle toward this person as you direct the same prayer phrases toward them for at least two full minutes:

May you have love (inhale).
May you have joy (exhale).
May you have peace (inhale).
May you have healing (exhale).
May you have rest (inhale).

Don't be surprised or come down hard on yourself if you immediately feel anger and resistance arise. Those are normal feelings. But I promise that if you faithfully practice this six-minute exercise every morning for the next four weeks, you will miraculously feel your heart open and change toward the person who wounded you. You will no longer feel the same negative emotional charge when their name comes up in conversations. You will find that God has mysteriously defrosted your heart, and you will want for them what you want for yourself—namely, peace, freedom, happiness, and flourishment.

The Lexicon of Amends

We make amends to people we've hurt in order to free ourselves from the shackles of the past—the guilt, shame, and self-hatred we feel over our mistakes and behaviors that stoke our addictions and self-defeating tendencies. Listen, the truth is that we can't recover unless we confront and eliminate these corrosive emotions. Just as important, we want to free those we've harmed from daily having to carry the burdens of resentment, anger, confusion, and sadness that our wrongdoings caused them. Remember, our goal in recovery is to become truly useful to God and of service to our fellows. Our effort to reconcile with those we've injured is one of the ways we accomplish this goal.

Direct Amends

As it turns out, there's not just one but several different kinds of amends. The first and best kind takes place in a face-to-face conversation between you and the person you harmed. This is called a *direct amends*.

All of us know from firsthand experience that there's a right and wrong way to ask for forgiveness and make amends.

We know because at some point in our lives, we've been on the wrong end of a botched apology that ended up doing more harm than good. What I've been taught in my program of recovery is that making a proper direct amends includes these five steps. (Frankly, I can't understand why we don't teach this stuff to kids in elementary school. It should be part of the curriculum of life.)

Step One: Name It and Claim It

As the brilliant novelist Zadie Smith writes in the introduction to Toni Morrison's book *Recitatif*, "It's difficult to 'move on' from any site of suffering if that suffering goes unacknowledged and undescribed."[3] Thus the first thing we must do when we meet with a person we've hurt is look them in the eye, acknowledge and describe our wrongdoing, and express our regret. The person to whom we're making our amends needs to know that *we* know in no uncertain terms the exact nature and gravity of our misdeed and that we're remorseful. This is not the time for euphemisms or word games.

If you stole a person's wallet, say, "I stole your wallet, and I want to make things right," not, "It's possible that I might have permanently borrowed your wallet without consulting you." At this point, we must also tell the person that their feelings about what we did are entirely legitimate, as in, "I stole your wallet *and* you have every right to be furious and disappointed in me. I would be too. I hope you can forgive me."

Step Two: Make Space for the Other Person

Once we've named the harm we've caused and asked for forgiveness, we make space for the person to share their thoughts and feelings with us openly. We can't skip this step, no matter how uncomfortable it may be. Hearing and understanding how our misdeed affected the injured party is critical to an amends conversation. We need to let the person we hurt describe the impact our wrongdoing had on their lives and how it made them feel—*without interrupting them.*

The person we hurt will often ask what motivated us to do what we did, so we should come prepared to offer a brief and unvarnished explanation. You might be tempted at this juncture to reframe, minimize, justify, or rationalize your poor behavior. For the love of all that is good, don't! The goal is to clear up the offended person's understandable confusion about what led you to violate or hurt them so they don't have to ruminate about it for the rest of time. Thus, a good explanation might be, "I stole your wallet because I was selfish and needed money to buy beer or a new game console."

Step Three: Let Them Add

When the harmed person appears to have finished sharing their thoughts and feelings, ask if they have anything else they'd like to add. If they don't, you should propose an appropriate amends, such as "I'd like to replace your wallet and pay you back the money I stole from it." It is also suggested that you ask the person if your proposed amends is acceptable to them or if you need to do something further to remedy the pain and suffering you caused them and to repair the breach in your relationship.

Step Four: Describe Your Future Intention

An amends that doesn't include a sincere commitment not to repeat the offending behavior isn't an amends; it's a juke.

You must promise you will not repeat your misdeed, as in, "From this day forward, I vow never again to steal your wallet or anything else from you."

Step Five: Go and Sin No More!

According to Merriam-Webster, the word *amend* means "to change or modify (something) for the better." We finish our amends by making a genuine commitment to "go and sin no more" (John 8:11 NLT), or at least not nearly as often as we did in the past. Of course, we aren't perfect. We will stumble. But we promise to give it our best shot. Remember, we seek progress, not perfection.

Indirect Amends

But what if we can't make a direct amends because the person we harmed lives five thousand miles away, or we haven't seen them for years or can't locate them? Or worse yet, what if they're dead? In this case, we make *indirect amends*.

In the case of the people we can't find, we pray that God will choreograph a "coincidental" meetup with them one day. My friend Barbara prayed this prayer about a long-lost friend she had hurt in her season of active addiction. Twenty years later, she ran into her estranged friend in the Qantas Lounge at the airport in Sydney, Australia, of all places. The two of them sat down, and Barbara made her amends. As they parted, they wished each other well. All this, and she didn't miss her connection to Los Angeles. "Good on ya, God," as the Aussies say.

Needless to say, making an indirect amends to a person who has died poses a unique challenge, but it's not impossible. The first time I got sober, my father had just died and I didn't have the chance to make a direct amends to him. My then-sponsor Greg suggested I write a letter to my dad that acknowledged the ways I had failed him, asked for his forgiveness, and shared with him my plans to live differently moving forward in his absence. When I finished the letter, Greg and I drove to the cemetery where my father is buried, and I stood at the foot of his grave and read my amends aloud to him. It was a powerful moment of healing and, more importantly for me, closure.

We also may have people on our amends list who are still too angry with us and will refuse to meet. In this instance, we pray that their hearts will eventually gentle toward us and we will one day have the chance to make a reparation. In the meantime, we can make an indirect amends to the person by performing a kindness we know would please or honor them. My friend Adam made indirect amends to a woman who told him never to contact her again by making an anonymous donation to the charity she worked for. Again, we do the best we can to sweep our side of the street.

Partial Amends

Step Nine comes with a caveat. It instructs us not to make any amends that would injure others. For example, a guy I met in treatment had a longstanding secret crush on his wife's best friend. When preparing to make amends to his wife for his many failures, he wondered if he should confess this to her. After praying about it and speaking to his sponsor, he discerned that it would cause more harm than good to tell her. Not only would it unnecessarily hurt his wife, but it would also potentially tarnish her relationship with her best friend, who hadn't done anything wrong. The point is, you don't want to unburden your conscience at the expense of another person's peace of mind.

A Few Tips

1. Be as calm and clear as you can during the amends conversation, and extend compassion to the person you harmed and to yourself. You both need it.
2. Keep things simple. Don't dive too deeply into all the facts and details surrounding your misdeeds, lest you resurface the pain in the person to whom you are making restitution. We're trying to heal people, not retraumatize them.
3. Whatever you do, do not bring up the other person's mistakes. This is about *your* misdeeds, not theirs.
4. When making your amends, you might become tearful, but try not to lose control of your emotions or start groveling and scraping. It's bad if the person you're making amends to has to hit pause on the conversation to comfort *you*. Be an adult. No one wants to see or hear from your inner crybaby right now.

Necessary Endings

Many, if not most, of your amends conversations will end well. You will be surprised at how kind and gracious other people can be when you humbly come clean with them and make a genuine effort to make restitution for your being a selfish prat. Some people won't remember the incident in question or won't think it was as big of a deal as you do. Others might say they admire you and ask how they can help you on your recovery journey. One of my first amends was to my friend Kathy, who I had hurt professionally in my active addiction. When I finished making my amends to her, she smiled and said, "Way to be a good human. Now buy me lunch at Ladybird Taco and I'll forget about it."

That said, it's possible that not all of your amends meetings will conclude on a happy note. My friend Dylan is a recovering porn and sex addict. When he went to his ex-wife to make amends to her, she told him there was nothing he could ever say or do that would repair the harm he had caused her. If this happens, the program tells us not to despair, but to remind ourselves that we did the best we could to right our wrongs and to accept the outcome. People have a right to be angry and not forgive us. Our primary goal isn't to heal the relationship (though that would be ideal), but rather to clean house so we're not tempted to drink, drug, or whatever to numb our unresolved guilt over previous misdeeds.

The best we can do when this happens is regularly pray for the healing of the person we harmed and that the day might come when we would be restored to a relationship with them. Then it's time to forgive ourselves and move forward. As Alice Munro wrote, "Moments of kindness and reconciliation are worth having, even if the parting has to come sooner or later."[4]

How to Make an Amends to Yourself

Finally, I asked my wife, Anne, to read my list and tell me if I had forgotten anyone. "I don't see your name on this list,"

Anne said, leafing through the pages. "Don't you think you should make amends to yourself for the way you've treated yourself?" At that moment I realized I had unknowingly put my name on my "Heck, no, I'll never make amends to that schmuck" list.

We all have a mental image of our ideal self against which we measure ourselves. Of course, this ideal self is unachievable and, therefore, tortures us. I'm not a full-blown perfectionist, but I have a finger-wagging schoolmaster who lives in my head. I call him the dean of admissions because I've given him the power to decide whether or not I'm worthy of entrance into the land of the forgiven. This is important. In your active addiction or compulsive behavior, you have no doubt hurt yourself as much as, or more than, you have others. You will have to forgive and make amends to yourself as you make genuine amends to others.

There is a passage in *The Big Book* at the end of the instructions for doing the Ninth Step that describes what we can expect to experience once we've made progress on our list. The passage is called "the ninth step promises," and it always moves me:

> If we are painstaking about this phase of our development, we will be amazed before we are half way through. We are going to know a new freedom and a new happiness. We will not regret the past nor wish to shut the door on it. We will comprehend the word *serenity* and we will know peace. No matter how far down the scale we have gone, we will see how our experience can benefit others. That feeling of uselessness and self-pity will

disappear. We will lose interest in selfish things and gain interest in our fellows. Self-seeking will slip away. Our whole attitude and outlook upon life will change. Fear of people and of economic insecurity will leave us. We will intuitively know how to handle situations which used to baffle us. We will suddenly realize that God is doing for us what we could not do for ourselves.[5]

Read these words before and after every amends you make. This is what you have to look forward to. Now, carry on!

Chapter Ten

LOOK OUT!

Spirituality means waking up.

Anthony de Mello, *Awareness*

STEP TEN

Continued to take personal inventory and when we were wrong promptly admitted it.

Recently, I read an article about two pilots who reportedly fell asleep in the cockpit while flying from New York City to Rome. Air traffic controllers frantically attempted to reach them for ten minutes, but there was no answer. Amid fears that terrorists had hijacked the Airbus A330 with 250 passengers on board, the tower was preparing to push out military jets to intercept the plane when the pilots finally woke up and responded.[1] *Surely, this doesn't happen very often*, I thought, tittering and trawling the internet for more information on the niche subject of somnolent pilots. But then I happened upon another article that said 56 percent of pilots admit to dozing off, and 29 percent report waking up to find their copilot sleeping.[2]

For antsy flyers like me, this is unwelcome news. In the words of aviation analyst John Nance, "The plane can still fly on autopilot, but this is not smart or safe."[3] John has a keen sense of the obvious.

As in aviation, so in life. For millennia, wise spiritual teachers have taught that human beings tend to fly through life spiritually asleep. We operate mostly on autopilot, blithely unaware of what we're doing or why. Obviously, falling asleep at the helm of our lives isn't smart. Heck, it's not safe for anybody. We need to *wake up*!

Wake Up!

As I've said previously, the purpose of the Twelve Steps is to facilitate a spiritual awakening that renders our need for numbing addictive substances or behaviors unnecessary and enables us to become emotionally and spiritually wiser people who can be of maximum service to God and others.

As we practice the Steps, our awareness of what God is up to in the moment expands and we become better equipped to align our thoughts, feelings, and actions with his will for us. We start living mindfully rather than mindlessly. We wake up!

If you're like me, however, you know from experience that it's easy to fall back asleep spiritually. Sometimes, your inner spiritual GPS loses its connection to the satellite and you find yourself lost and sleepwalking through emotionally sketchy neighborhoods. Step Ten is the solution!

Steps Ten through Twelve are called "the maintenance Steps" because they support our new way of life. In Steps One through Three, we made peace with God. In Steps Four through Seven, we made peace with ourselves. And in Steps Eight and Nine, we made peace with others. We've set our house in order. Now, in Steps Ten through Twelve, we create a lifestyle that maintains our new way of life.

Step Ten teaches us how to deftly tread through the

minefield of everyday life without reverting to our old knee-jerk addictions or loops of self-defeating behavior.

When I began working on Step Ten, it enabled me to face the little (and not so little) crises of daily life with equanimity—emotional balance in the face of whatever life threw my way. Bill Wilson called this grounded, awakened inner state "emotional sobriety,"[4] and it's blissful when you're in the flow of it.

Step Ten is what we do when we realize that there's a "disruption in the Force." For example, we've had an unhappy encounter with someone, which has thrown us off-kilter emotionally. How do we get back on the beam once we've fallen off it? The poet Rumi asks a vital question: "Do you pay regular visits to *yourself*?"[5] During these "regular visits," we use an abbreviated or slightly modified version of the personal inventory we first learned in Step Four to restore us to sanity. In fact, if practiced well, Step Ten is like repeating Steps Four through Nine all in one fell swoop!

There are at least three ways to take a personal inventory:

- the mental spot-check inventory, which can happen several times a day
- the written spot-check inventory
- the nightly inventory

I'm not a "*Big Book* thumper" or a Twelve-Step fundamentalist who claims "there's only one right way to do the Steps." Honestly, I know very few people who do all of these inventories every single day, but I think it's best to work all three of them in the beginning. Over time, you can customize this Step so it fits your needs and lifestyle. Before we jump into the nuts and bolts of how to perform these different inventories, let me introduce you to someone I hope will become your new best friend—your Inner Observer.

The Inner Observer

To live a happy, spiritually enlightened life, you need to awaken and daily rely on your Inner Observer (a.k.a. the seat of your self-awareness) for self-insight and guidance. When performing its job properly, your Inner Observer will watch your life like a movie and help you regulate your thoughts, feelings, and actions in real time as you go through the day. Your Inner Observer is like a life coach that actually knows what it's talking about and helps you remain awake and at the helm of your behaviors. It lets you know when your character defects have resurfaced, and how to go about restoring balance and calm.

Trust me, you don't want to leave home without your Inner Observer. When your Inner Observer is untrained or goes offline, you lose self-awareness. You begin operating on autopilot. Folks who lack self-awareness corner you at cocktail parties and say things that make you want to stick a toothpick in your eye so you have an excuse to go to the ER and escape their company. To live a spiritually attuned, emotionally intelligent, and serene life, you absolutely need the help of your Inner Observer.

I love my Inner Observer. He smiles and says things to me like, "Look at you, being all impatient again, blaring your car horn and yelling at people as if you believe this behavior will make a ten-mile-long traffic travesty magically disappear. Let's try responding instead of reacting, shall we? Take a few deep breaths and treat this unplanned delay as a gift, as an opportunity to pray for people or to make a few calls to encourage friends. That would make you a better citizen of the world right now, wouldn't it?"

Furthermore, no one asks me better questions than my Inner Observer. "What's coming up for you right now? Are you presently operating from a place of love or from a place of fear? Are you projecting one of your own faults onto that person and then punishing them for having it? Did you notice that your friend looked forlorn when you asked him about his marriage a few minutes ago? Maybe you should circle back and ask if he's okay."

Though my Inner Observer periodically questions my sanity—as in, "Tell me again why you think hitting Send on that blistering email to your condo association is a good idea right now?"—it also frequently catches me doing things right and congratulates me: "Heigh-ho! Did I just see you *not* lecture your adult child on what you think they should do with the rest of their lives? Well done, you!"

One of the more important things your Inner Observer will repeatedly tell you to do is take a pause. I was a hyperreactive person before I started working a Twelve-Step program. Honestly, I used to react to life like a guy trapped inside a phone booth with a murder hornet. I flapped and swatted at almost everything. It was exhausting. Then I happened upon an anonymous quote often attributed to the psychiatrist and author Viktor Frankl: "Between stimulus and response there is a space. In that space is our power to choose our response. In our response lies our growth and our freedom." My Inner Observer frequently whispers to me, "Easy does it. No need to immediately do or say something you will likely regret ten minutes from now. Pause, step into the space, and calmly consider what would be the most loving thing to do next."

Obviously, your Inner Observer is responsible for helping you perform inventories on your behavior in real time all day long. If it tells you to take a pause (a practice that *The Big Book* recommends numerous times!) before you speak or act, do it.

Spot-Check Inventory

Now on to the actual Tenth Step Inventories. Every day, we're given ample opportunity to make a mess of things. As my friend Matt says, "I could screw up a free cup of coffee." What do we do when an annoying situation arises or a triggering interaction hijacks us?

I'm not always great at rising to the moment. Several mornings a week, I visit my favorite cafe on Nashville's historic Music Row to treat myself to a cortado. Usually, this is a happy outing, but on the morning in question, I was feeling poorly. It was August in Tennessee. My sweat-drenched clothes were shellacked to my body; my bad knee was cranky with me; and I was racing against the clock to meet a writing deadline. As my elderly neighbor Miss Gladys used to say, "I was fixin' to pitch a hissy fit."

When I arrived at the café, I discovered a bubbly new barista was having long, giggly conversations with every customer in line, even though the queue for drinks was out the door. I overheard her tell one of the customers that her name was Felicity. *Figures*, I thought, rolling my eyes. Like I said, I was in a mood.

When it came to my turn in line, Felicity smiled at me like she was rushing me to join her sorority. "What can I make you, hon?" she asked.

"A cortado," I said curtly, looking at my watch.

"How would you like it?" she said.

"I'd like it *today*," I replied icily.

Felicity's smile vanished, and her eyes narrowed. Several minutes later, when she handed me my cortado, she muttered, "Have a blessed day, jackass."

Furious, I stormed out of the café and immediately called Sponsor Steve from the car and told him what had gone down at my coffee stop. "Do you think this might be an opportunity to practice a Tenth Step?" he offered.

This is precisely why I hate Sponsor Steve. I wanted him to hop on my resentment wagon and trash-mouth the terminally cheerful Felicity, but instead, he turned all "A.A.-Jesus" on me and suggested I go back and make nice with her. As I've said, Sponsor Steve is right more often than he's wrong, so I pulled a U-ey and drove back to the café.

When I arrived, the line was gone, and Felicity was wiping down the counters. "Hi," I said. "I was here a few minutes ago and acted like an idiot. I just wanted to come back and ask your forgiveness. Can I make it up to you somehow?"

"Oh my gosh," Felicity gushed, running out from behind the counter to hug me. "I'm sorry too! When you left, I realized I was still angry from an argument I'd had with my boyfriend this morning, and I dumped all that negative energy on you!"

The clouds parted; the sun shone. Felicity and I were in couples' therapy. We were having a moment. In that brief exchange, I learned Felicity had recently moved to Nashville from Idaho Springs, Colorado, to become a songwriter, that her soon-to-be ex-boyfriend was a useless couch lump, and she dreamt of one day owning a hairless cat. Ten minutes later, I walked out the door with a happy heart and a free double shot cortado with extra cinnamon. The universe winked at me. My day was looking up.

On the drive home, I texted Sponsor Steve: "I have a new best friend. Her name is Felicity."

In *Twelve Steps and Twelve Traditions*, Bill Wilson writes, "It is a spiritual axiom that every time we are disturbed, no matter what the cause, there is something wrong *with us*."[6] I hated that sentence when I first read it. *Surely, it's not always my fault when things go wrong and I get angry or resentful at someone*, I thought. But this recognition and acceptance of personal responsibility is good news. It means I'm not a passive victim of circumstances. I can own my inner turmoil and do something about it.

What I did with Felicity is called a "mental spot-check inventory." I felt disturbed. I checked in with a friend. I mentally reviewed and owned my less-than-mature reaction to the situation. I cleaned up after myself. This isn't quantum physics, folks. It's what my kids call "adulting."

But what do I do when I have a lava-hot, tooth-jarring encounter with someone? In that case, more than a mental spot-check inventory might be required. I need something more, so I will quickly pull out my journal and *write out* my spot-check inventory. When we put our thoughts and feelings to paper, we see things we previously hadn't seen, and we gain perspective. Had I done this in the case of Felicity versus Cron, my journal entry would have read:

I'm resentful at: Felicity

Why: She wasn't performing her job to my satisfaction, and she called me a jackass.

How did it affect me? My interaction with Felicity bruised my pride and offended my tetchy ego.

What was my part? I wasn't in touch with my Inner Observer, and I reacted rather than responded. I behaved like an entitled two-year-old and spoke unkindly.

What could I have done differently: I could have paused, taken a breath, cut Felicity a little slack, and been more tolerant and loving. She was only trying to be friendly to her customers.

What should I do now? Be a good lad and go back and make amends to Felicity.

We can also perform a quick spot-check inventory when we have an emotional hiccup that doesn't involve another person, like when an unpleasant feeling surfaces unbidden. It's hard to admit, but I regularly compare myself to others and feel envious. Not long ago, I was driving through a posh neighborhood in Nashville and began to think, *Wait a minute. I'm a smart guy. Why don't I live in one of these big houses? Don't I deserve to have a Range Rover in my driveway, fly on private jets, and own a summer cottage in the Hamptons?*

I know, my occasional flights into entitlement make my hair hurt too. Thankfully, my Inner Observer picked up on the emotional charge of envy rising in my chest and cued me to perform a mental spot-check inventory to untangle myself from it. Here's how it went:

What's happening: I'm driving past beautiful homes and feeling resentful that I'm not better off than I am.

What's it affecting: This line of thinking embarrasses me.

What's my part: I'm prone to envy and not being grateful for my amazing life.

What should I do now? Stop whining, call my friend Graham to tell him about my crazy thinking, have a good laugh, and make a gratitude list.

You know what happens when you perform a mental or written spot-check inventory, right? You wake up.

Nightly Inventory

The Big Book also encourages us to nightly review how our day went, what we learned, where we succeeded, and where we need to improve; to set goals for the next day; and, if necessary, to plan to make amends. In a perfect world, I would be able to instantly notice every time I screw up and immediately take care of it, but I can't. This is why a nightly inventory is important.

If you hop on the internet and search "nightly Tenth Step inventory" you'll find a million worksheets, tutorials, apps, and suggestions on how to perform one. Remember, there's no single right way to do the steps. That said, here's how I do mine. Before I turn out the light and go to sleep, I grab my journal, chronologically review the day, and answer these questions (some people prefer to do this exercise mentally, while others choose to write out the answers; because I tend to fall asleep whenever I close my eyes, I prefer the latter):

1. Was I resentful?
2. Was I dishonest?
3. Did I promptly admit when I was wrong?
4. Do I owe anyone an apology or amends?
5. Did I do or say something out of fear?
6. Have I kept something to myself that should be discussed with another person immediately?
7. Did I think today of what I could do for others?
8. Was I kind and loving toward all?
9. Did I reach out to someone in recovery today to ask how they were doing?
10. What could I have done better?

A miracle of my recovery is that I'm able to make inventories without shaming or beating myself up when I find I wasn't at my best that day. My Inner Observer is not an Inner Critic.

The Periodic Whole Life Inventory

Lots of folks I know in recovery book an overnight at a monastery or beach house for an annual or biannual retreat to do a more comprehensive housecleaning inventory. These are wonderful opportunities to meditate, pray, and take honest stock of our spiritual, emotional, physical, social, and professional lives. Most people avoid self-appraisal and pay a price for it. It's called mediocrity . . . at best.

One of my favorite stories comes from author Gregory Knox Jones. Many years ago, the British came up with the idea of building a golf course in Calcutta, India. This was an ambitious project that required a great deal of planning and labor. When construction of the course was complete, the British were very, very pleased with themselves. But when the first flight of golfers teed off, the players realized there was a contingency the engineers had failed to bake into their calculations—monkeys.

Every time a player hit a ball, a pack of laughing monkeys would run out onto the fairway, grab the rolling ball, and throw it in all directions. At first, the British tried shooing the monkeys away. When that didn't work, they built a tall fence around the course, but the monkeys climbed over it. Exasperated, the British tried capturing and relocating the monkeys, but there were just too many of them. Finally, the British came up with a brilliant solution. They established a rule they wrote into the club's playbook. It read, "You have to play the ball where the monkey drops it."[7]

Not a week goes by when I don't repeat that clever rule to myself at least once. Life presents us with a difficult syllabus. To live happily, we need to be adaptable, cultivate resilience, and regularly practice self-reflection.

Regularly taking Step Ten will teach you to accept and work with your life as it is, even when you don't like where the monkey dropped the ball. It will help you recognize where you are on your spiritual path and which shot you have to play next to improve your game. Reflecting on Step Ten, Bill Wilson wrote, "For the wise have always known that no one can make much of his life until self-searching becomes a regular habit, until he is able to admit and accept what he finds, and until he patiently and persistently tries to correct what is wrong."[8]

Trust me, you will experience such remarkable benefits from taking regular time to examine your inner world that you will eventually look forward to it.

Chapter Eleven

SO HELP ME GOD

Dear Jesus, do something.

Vladimir Nabokov, *Pale Fire*

STEP ELEVEN

Sought through prayer and meditation to improve our conscious contact with God as we understood Him, praying only for knowledge of His will and the power to carry that out.

My favorite game as a kid was hide-and-seek, perhaps because I'm genetically optimized for it. More flexible than a carnival contortionist, I could twist my pint-sized frame into shapes and positions that allowed me to squeeze into unimaginably tight places where people never bothered to look.

But I soon learned a hard lesson—being a great hider is no fun. No one could ever find me. I once hid in a cereal box–sized wicker hamper for an hour before realizing that my friends had given up searching for me and moved on to Wiffle ball. Where's the whoopee in that?

While in rehab, I had an epiphany—I brought my talent for concealment into adulthood. I'm an expert at hiding not only from people but from God and myself too. Shame and fear are cruel and unrelenting bullies, aren't they? What prudent person wants to risk discovery and exposure when experience tells you it will only lead to ridicule and rejection?

There are lots of clever places where grownups can hide themselves. We hide behind the drapes of our achievements, under our educational degrees, beneath the facade of our impressive résumés, inside our safe but uncritically accepted religious convictions, behind blustery or meek personas, atop the towers of our soaring intellects, and behind the mask of our often calculated vulnerability. You name it. Anything can be a wicker hamper if you want it to be.

Our addictions are a hiding place as well, right? We crawl into them to hide from the ceaseless demands of life, to numb the Big Ache, to distract ourselves from our anxiety, self-doubt, and depressions—as if a quick hit of sugar, a third bourbon, or the long-awaited smile of appreciation will return us to the warm safety of the womb. But guess what? What's true in hide-and-seek is true in the spiritual life—it's no fun if you're too good at hiding. In the divine game of hide-and-seek, the point is to let God find you.

But how does someone who has spent a lifetime concealing themselves learn to live in the open?

Prayer

Bill Wilson believed prayer and meditation were the practices best suited to help people emerge from behind their masks and addictions and improve their conscious contact with God. I would be surprised if a few of us weren't feeling slightly disappointed right now. "Not prayer and meditation again! Surely there must be more exciting, less analog ways to draw closer to the heart of God than those old chestnuts!" If you feel this way (and I sympathize if you do), then perhaps you need to reimagine what prayer and meditation are.

As a little kid, my parents and teachers inadvertently taught me that prayer was transactional. I begged and bargained with God to give me what I wanted, tacked on a few Hail Marys, and went on with my day, hoping for the best. But grownup prayer isn't nudging or bumping God's arm with your nose and pleadingly staring at him until he begrudgingly gives in and satisfies the pettish demands of our egos. That's what your poodle does to you when it wants a treat.

In real prayer, we seek to quiet the demands of our self-centered egos and seek peaceful alignment with God's purpose for our lives, no matter what that entails. "Let go and let God," as Twelve-Step old-timers say. For me, the whole point of prayer is to "undergo his presence" as Father Ronald Rolheiser writes,[1] to achieve union with God, until you one day find that his thoughts, feelings, and desires are precisely the same as yours.

In *The Big Book*, Bill Wilson repeatedly urges his recovering readers to recite what I've come to believe is the "Big Mama" of all prayers: "Thy will be done."[2] Now if you're old enough to vote, you've lived long enough to know that this is a seriously dangerous prayer. It involves telling your Prada-clad ego to take a number (other than the number 1) and go stand at the back of the line.

Praying and living the words "Thy will be done" are radical acts of self-surrender. Adopting an open-handed posture toward life, to truly accept life on life's terms, requires courage, discipline, and no small amount of effort. It's the spiritual equivalent of climbing Everest in penny loafers and without supplemental oxygen. To reach the summit and stay sober, you're going to need serious high-tech gear—namely, prayer and meditation.

Now remember, Step Eleven is one of the maintenance Steps (Ten though Twelve) that I mentioned in the previous chapter. By now, your journey through the Steps has facilitated a healing in the rupture of your relationship with God (One through Three), yourself (Four through Seven), and with others (Eight and Nine). In Step Ten, you made a commitment to cultivate self-awareness and correct your mistakes as they happen. As part of your maintenance program (Ten through Twelve), Step Eleven offers you tools to stay connected to the Source.

Be forewarned, if you skip or shortchange Step Eleven, your program will be built on willful self-propulsion, which, no matter how well-intentioned it may be, will ultimately fail you. Remember, you're powerless, and you won't overcome your addictions, recurrent self-defeating behaviors, and character defects, or become like Jesus through your own unaided strength or on your own terms. If you try, you will become discouraged and give up, or, worse yet, you will clothe yourself in the veneer of Christian piety and become a pious religious prig like Mrs. Turpin in Flannery O'Connor's short story "Revelation."[3] Please don't do this—the world already has enough of these breathing annoyances.

Now, to mechanics.

The How of Prayer

My friend Mary's former sponsor Bob used to end every conversation with her by saying, "Remember, you're brain-broke." Bob's wry reminder might sound a wee bit Eeyore-ish, but I get his gist. My brain is a dangerous place for me to wander alone in without adult supervision. If I don't set aside time to pray and stay connected to God, I will corkscrew into a hot mess. I know from experience that if I don't begin every day on my knees and lash myself to God, it's "Katy bar the door!" time.

As I mentioned earlier, I'm a Christian of the Episcopal persuasion. If you let me freestyle pray for too long, I'm apt to discursively ramble on about a wide swath of topics, ranging from who I want as our next president to worrying aloud about my fear of contracting tropical jungle rot. That's why I like liturgy—set prayers and an "order of service." Why reinvent the prayer wheel when the Bible and *The Big Book* are full of perfectly worded, time-tested beauties? And so I've put together my own morning recovery prayer liturgy, loosely based on the "Daily Devotions for Individuals and Families" found in *The Book of Common Prayer.*[4]

As you'll see, my morning prayer time includes the same elements and follows the same pattern every day. It includes Scripture-based prayers, spiritual readings, journaling, recovery prayers, spontaneous prayers, and meditation.

Though it may sound like my morning meetup with God is overfull and would take me until lunchtime to complete, it's not as onerous as it sounds. I can usually get it done in thirty minutes. Here's an example:

Opening prayer from Psalm 51:[5]

Open my lips, O Lord,
and my mouth shall proclaim your praise.
Create in me a clean heart, O God,
and renew a right spirit within me.

Cast me not away from your presence
and take not your holy Spirit from me.
Give me the joy of your saving help again
and sustain me with your bountiful Spirit.
Glory to the Father, and to the Son, and to the Holy Spirit:
as it was in the beginning, is now, and will be for ever. Amen.

Spiritual reading: Here I read a short passage from Scripture or a chapter from a book about living the spiritual life or fostering personal development.

Gratitude journal: The torchlight of my attention tends to focus its beam on what's not working or what's absent in my life rather than on what is working or is present. To cultivate a positive, abundance mindset, I daily write down at least three things I'm grateful for in my life and recovery.

Twenty-minute silent meditation: Humans are strange creatures. We'll willingly spend an hour standing in a milelong line in 100-degree heat just for the thrill of a nausea-inducing three-minute roller-coaster ride at Walt Disney World, but we recoil when someone suggests we spend a few minutes each day silently resting in the love of God. Listen, no other spiritual practice has given me so much for doing so little. More on this in a moment!

Prayers for others: This is where I pray specifically for friends, family, the state of the world, and myself.

Deliver me prayer:

From the need of being praised, deliver me, Jesus.
From the need of being honored, deliver me, Jesus.
From the need of being preferred, deliver me, Jesus.

From the need of being consulted, deliver me, Jesus.

From the need of being approved, deliver me, Jesus.

From the need of being right, deliver me, Jesus.

From the need of comfort and ease, deliver me, Jesus.

From the fear of being humiliated, deliver me, Jesus.

From the fear of being criticized, deliver me, Jesus.

From the fear of being passed over, deliver me, Jesus.

From the fear of being forgotten, deliver me, Jesus.

From the fear of being lonely, deliver me, Jesus.

From the fear of being hurt, deliver me, Jesus.

From the fear of suffering, deliver me, Jesus.

O Jesus, help me put my self-importance aside.

O Jesus, make my heart like yours.

O Jesus, strengthen me with your Spirit.

O Jesus, teach me your ways.

Amen.

"Litany of Humility," adapted from a prayer by
Rafael Cardinal Merry del Val, 1865–1930

Closing prayer:[6]

Lord God, almighty and everlasting Father, you have brought us in safety to this new day: Preserve us with your mighty power, that we may not fall into sin, nor be overcome by adversity; and in all we do, direct us to the fulfilling of your purpose; through Jesus Christ our Lord. Amen.

And that's it.

You might be thinking, *Ian, you actually do the same thing every day?* Yes. Like a golfer who hits ball after ball at the driving range, I believe in the power of repetition. I want to reach a point where I repeat set prayers often enough that they eventually work themselves into my bones and blood, and maybe, just maybe, I will one day *become* the prayer itself. I'm building spiritual muscle memory.

All the elements in my morning recovery liturgy are essential, but two are worth highlighting. As you now know, the ego is never satisfied. It always feels deprived. All day long, it shrieks, "Feed me!" like the ever-starving, man-eating plant Audrey II in the Broadway musical *Little Shop of Horrors*. It never gets precisely what it wants, and whatever it wants, it wants it *now*. This is why keeping a gratitude journal is so important for me.

Few things will quiet, gladden, and rightsize my chattering ego like cataloging a few of the many kindnesses God regularly bestows on me. As Bill Wilson wrote, "I try hard to hold fast to the truth that a full and thankful heart cannot entertain great conceits. When brimming with gratitude, one's heartbeat must surely result in outgoing love, the finest emotion that we can ever know."[7]

As I mentioned earlier, I make a point of writing down a minimum of three items in my gratitude journal every day. When Sponsor Steve first encouraged me to begin this discipline, I dismissed it as a quaint but probably useless thing to do, but over time, this practice has produced a radical transformation in how I see and relate to the world. Now whether I'm prowling around the house feeling "irritable, restless, and discontented"[8] or just happily traipsing down the street, I find myself reflexively pausing to express gratitude for even the "small things"—my dogs, coffee, clementines, and cashmere (I'm allergic to wool). Finally, in my gratitude journaling, I always include a problem or challenge that's currently teaching me something important. As Paula D'Arcy wrote, "God comes to you disguised as your life."[9] Thus, we should try to be grateful for our real and seeming hardships as well.

Finally, as a person in recovery, I know about the perils of cross addictions. Like a crazy-eyed mob of Black Friday shoppers, there are plenty of other addictions waiting to crash through the doors of my life and take me hostage. This is why I regularly review my life to see if I'm falling prey to other addictions or compulsions that are beginning to compete for my loyalty to God. And so I write this formula in my journal: "God, help me find in you what I look for in _____." I want to confront and surrender any addictive substance or behavior (e.g., money, people-pleasing, work, overeating, compulsively checking my iPhone, and so forth) that stands between me and realizing union with God.

The When of Prayer

You can converse with God wherever, however, and as often as you like (preferably a lot). God is not proud. He doesn't care if you want to commune with him while swimming, hiking, walking your corgis, dancing to old Eminem records, or making box lanyards with the kids. Like the seventeenth-century Carmelite lay monk Brother Lawrence, I aspire to become a person who "practices the presence of God" at all times, whether folding my socks or clattering away on my computer writing a book. In short, I'm training myself to stay connected to God 24-7 through my prayer practice.

Okay, so now we've discussed conscious, spoken prayer.

But what do we do with the shadowy, hidden drives; fiery longings; and troublesome phantoms that unconsciously govern our lives for which we have no words? How can we give God access to our innermost selves and allow him to heal the unseen, broken places in our adumbral depths?

It is dangerous to presume you know yourself better than you do. You know only a tiny fraction of yourself. The unconscious (what the Bible calls your *heart*) is a vast, mysterious country littered with all kinds of crazy emotional and psychological trash that needs regularly taking out. This shouldn't surprise us. We think, speak, dream, and do things all the time that spook us. These curious and often harmful thoughts and behaviors arise from the unconscious, and there's much we can't change about ourselves unless we grant God access into our "inner rooms" to do his thing.

We have little access to this dark province of madness and the mess it contains, and even if we could enter it, we'd have no clue how to set things in order. As I've often heard it said, "No problem can be solved from the same level of consciousness that created it," and that's spot-on. So, what do we do?

Glad you asked. It's time to talk about meditation.

Meditation

Some Christians break out in hives when they hear the word *meditation*. It conjures up the image of a Buddhist yogi sitting atop an elephant as the yogi holds a lotus flower, chanting, "Om." I understand. But listen, meditation has a long and storied history in the Christian tradition. The desert mothers and fathers practiced a form of it as far back as the third century. So don't think that if you adopt a meditation practice, you'll wake up one day in an Indian ashram, wondering, *Oh my, how did I get* here? Breathe. Be open-minded. It'll be alright.

Five months after I returned home from rehab, I attended a weeklong, silent meditation retreat in Asheville, North Carolina. I had long had a fascination with meditation. Over the years, I had read stacks of books about the history and practice of meditation in the Christian and Buddhist traditions. I'd gone down the wormhole of studying secular research about the evidence-based, psychological benefits of practicing mindfulness. More importantly, I knew that Bill Wilson strongly suggested meditation as a vital spiritual tool, and many of my friends from "the rooms" testified to how valuable it has been in their programs of recovery. In other words, I knew a lot about meditation and its importance, at least in theory. All that remained for me was to actually *do* it.

While waiting in line at the registration table, I picked up and perused the outline of the daily schedule. When I read that we would be spending six hours a day in silent meditation, I nearly had a heart attack. Sure, there were breaks for instruction, eating plant-based meals (e.g., vegan carrot "hot dogs" on gluten-free spinach buns), and doing early morning yoga, but otherwise we would be sitting silently with our eyes closed, trying to quiet our minds and focus on a "sacred word" for *six hours* a day. I was aghast. I can't sit still for five minutes, let alone six hours. *What about blood clots?* I wondered. What nearly drove me over the edge is when I learned the retreat center dining hall served only decaf coffee. *This isn't a retreat center; it's a gulag,* I thought. *What have I done?*

Though physically, emotionally, and spiritually challenging, the retreat turned out to be one of the most important weeks of my life. During that time, I learned and practiced centering prayer, or what Julian of Norwich called "oneing with God."[10] The inspiration for centering prayer is drawn from the Matthew 6:6: "When you pray, go into your room, close the door and pray to your Father, who is unseen. Then your Father, who sees what is done in secret, will reward you."

The purpose of centering prayer is to silently usher us into the presence of God, where we surrender and offer him permission to enter our unconscious and rewire our "broke brains" and hearts. Father Thomas Keating, the pioneer of the modern centering prayer movement, calls centering prayer "divine therapy"[11]—and it's free of charge!

Thomas Merton wrote, "The greatest need of our time is to clean out the enormous mass of mental and emotional rubbish that clutters our minds."[12] Truer words have never been spoken. Addicts (us!) are cursed with monkey minds. Our thoughts and emotions leap limb to limb all day long. It makes your head hurt, right? The wonderful thing is you're not asked to think, feel, or say anything in centering prayer. In it, you discover the relative unimportance of words. God resides beyond their boundaries.

Okay, enough of this mystical, airy-fairy talk. Let's discuss technique. Here's how centering prayer works.[13]

1. Choose a sacred word. This word is a symbol of your intention "to consent to God's presence and action within." Your sacred word isn't a mantra but an anchor you'll repeatedly return to and focus on when

you catch yourself reengaging with your thoughts. Your sacred word could be *Jesus*, *love*, *present*, or my go-to—*shalom*. Some people use an abbreviated form of the Jesus Prayer: "Lord, have mercy on me." The phrase contains more words than you need, but as prayers go, it has a long and honorable history. Regardless, once you've chosen your word or short phrase, stick with it.

2. Sit in a comfortable position with your eyes closed, relax, and silently say your sacred word as "the symbol of your consent to God's presence and action within."

3. When your attention wanders (and it will!) and you start replaying an argument you had with your teen the night before or suddenly remember you need to pick up your dry cleaning, gently return to your sacred word until your mind quiets again. Then when your mind has calmed and repeating your sacred word is no longer necessary, let it go.

4. When you're finished, sit quietly for a few minutes and enjoy the afterglow of your time in God's presence. Then slowly open your eyes, get up, and fire up the espresso machine.

Now be careful. Centering prayer is so easy you're going to want to make it hard. You'll be tempted to play a little ambient music to get you in the mood, or you'll want to imagine yourself sitting by a river holding Jesus' hand to make the experience feel more spiritual while you're doing it. There's nothing wrong with doing these things per se—just that they won't help you. They're simply another form of monkey mind. The key is to disengage from your *terribly* interesting thoughts and mental pictures, empty yourself, and fall gently into God.

Father Keating suggested we could work toward having two twenty-minute meditation sessions a day—one in the morning and another in the late afternoon.[14] I know, that's crazy. I'm still only able to practice one sit a day. But I believe in you! I recommend you start with five minutes in the morning, and once that's comfortable, incrementally titrate the time to the recommended dose. Be patient. It may take a while.

If you're like me when I started, one thought that will repeatedly come up while you're practicing centering prayer is, *What's the point?*

Well, when you've practiced centering prayer for a few weeks you will begin to notice something amazing happening. You will naturally find yourself doing things you've been trying to do through your unaided strength all your life but have failed to accomplish on your own. You will feel more grounded and centered in God throughout the day. Your Inner Observer will awaken, and your ability to take a pause in heated moments will strengthen. You won't easily take offense, and you will become more loving, patient, and tolerant with yourself and other people. Your perceptive appreciation of the world will intensify, and feelings of awe and wonder will return. You will more easily laugh at yourself and maybe get misty-eyed watching your kids play in the yard, as if seeing them for the first time.

You will observe these changes and ask yourself, *How did this happen?* and then you'll realize that it's the fruit of your centering prayer practice. Through meditation, God is slowly changing you into the person you always wanted with hardly any effort on your part.

A recent experience revealed another fruit of my centering prayer practice. A few months ago, I found myself sitting across from a bespectacled, emotionally unresponsive pulmonologist who was squinting at an X-ray of my chest. My internist had already told me there was growing concern that I had a lung condition that might end my earthly pilgrimage much sooner than I had planned. I was more than a little on edge. While I waited for the pulmonologist to look up and deliver his verdict, I silently said, *God, help me, I'm scared. I want to grow old and see my grandkids.*

As is often the case, God's help came to me in an unexpected way. Sitting there, I suddenly remembered Bill Wilson's admonition in Step Eleven to pray "only for knowledge of his will for us and the power to carry that out."[15] Unconsciously, I found the words of my prayer changing from "Please don't let this be what they think it might be" to "God, I have no idea what you're up to right now, but I choose to believe that you're in charge. *Thy will be done.*"

I wish I could say this surprising about-face in my prayer from pleading to surrendering to God's will for my life, *no matter what*, happened because I'm a spiritual giant, but I can't. I believe the in-the-moment nudge from God to shift my spiritual perspective was a fruit of my showing up and suiting up for my daily oneing session with him. Beyond that, I did nothing. It was a grace. Thankfully, the ominous shadow on my lung X-ray turned out to be a false negative.

"Well, you can't end the story there, Ian," you might say. "What would your reaction have been if the X-ray result had come back positive for lung disease?" It's a good question, one I've thought long and hard about. I can't say for sure what my response would have been if I had been handed dire news, but I can tell you what I would like it to be.

That morning, on my way to the pulmonologist's office, I got a call from Sponsor Steve.

"How are you feeling?" Steve said, getting right to the point.

"I guess everything'll be okay," I said, in a voice that sounded more like a question than a firm conviction.

There was a long pause on the other end of the line. "Everything already is okay, Ian," Sponsor Steve said, the spiritual freight of his words falling on me like a pallet of bricks.

To believe that everything's okay, right now, no matter how bleak things appear, is where I'm aiming to go and how I want to be in the world. It's where Jesus finally arrived at Gethsemane when he surrendered, saying, "Yet not my will, but yours be done" (Luke 22:42). But only a lifelong practice of prayer and meditation can produce that kind of titanic faith and emotional sobriety. I'm not there yet. And so, until God tells me otherwise, I'm going to keep showing up to my meditation cushion every morning (or most mornings), saying my prayers, sipping a little *real* coffee, and waiting for the miracle.

Chapter Twelve

IT WORKS IF YOU WORK IT

You were sick, but now you're well again, and there's work to do.
Kurt Vonnegut, *Timequake*

STEP TWELVE

Having had a spiritual awakening as the result of these Steps, we tried to carry this message to alcoholics [our fellow sufferers], and to practice these principles in all our affairs.

A few months before my wife Anne's fortieth birthday, I asked her how she would like to celebrate her big day. "I want to run the Ocean State Marathon together in October," she said with a smile as she handed me a book titled *Four Months to a Four-Hour Marathon.*[1]

A wave of dread washed over me. As I've mentioned, Anne is a fit and fiercely competitive athlete, whereas my idea of exercise is "a good, brisk sit," as the old-school comedian Phyllis Diller once quipped.[2] How could I keep up with her for 26.2 miles? Not wanting to disappoint Anne, I accepted her challenge and wholeheartedly threw myself into a running regime that felt more like a death march than fitness training. I was actually beginning to feel like I could finish the marathon when disaster struck—two weeks before race day, I pulled my hamstring so severely that I could barely walk. But after enduring three months of grueling workouts, I was determined not to throw in the towel.

I immediately called my doctor, who advised me to go

to the pharmacy and buy a product called Icy Hot. If you're unfamiliar with it, Icy Hot is a mentholated ointment that penetrates the skin and soothes sore muscles. Like anyone with an addictive temperament, I operate under the assumption that "If a little is good, more must be better." And so, I scooped out half the jar of Icy Hot and slathered it on my hamstring.

Unbeknownst to me, however, while hiking up my running shorts, they brushed against the back of my thigh, and a continent-sized dollop of Icy Hot dislodged and smeared itself all over its inner lining—you know, the built-in underwear that ensures that your privates don't fall out while you're running. I then merrily set out on a ten-mile training run.

Looking back, I can see that my first mistake was not reading the directions on the jar. If I had, I would have learned the effects of Icy Hot intensify as your body temperature rises. And so, five miles into my run, I realized that a particularly delicate region of my anatomy was warming up and feeling "minty fresh." *That's a novel sensation,* I thought.

But after another mile and a continuing rise in body temperature, the sensation turned from "minty fresh" to alarmingly uncomfortable. Now I started to panic. *I'm six miles from home and experiencing a wardrobe malfunction involving fire. What should I do?* Tragically, the only idea I could come up with was to turn around and start sprinting. This was my second mistake. You see, the faster I ran, the more my body temperature increased, and the more my body temperature increased, the hotter the Icy Hot became . . . you see where this is heading, right?

Soon, my privates were ablaze. It was as if someone had poured an accelerant into my knickers. I was now in whimpering agony, scampering down the street with my hands in the fig leaf position. A car full of concerned-looking teens pulled alongside me and yelled out the open windows, "Do you need help, sir?" but I was in so much pain that I couldn't form a coherent sentence to answer them. All I could think about was getting home and plunging into a cold bath to extinguish the fire consuming my . . . well, you know.

When I turned the corner toward home, I saw my then three- and six-year-old daughters playing in the front yard. They thought I was joking around when they saw me sprinting down the street yelling, "Give way! Give way!" and they started giggling and running in circles, imitating me. However, they realized something was seriously amiss when I ran past them and through the front door, tearing off my running clothes. "Mommy, something's wrong with Daddy," they shrieked, running behind me into the house.

Yeah, my kids have had lots of therapy.

But my daughters were right. Something *was* wrong with Daddy. He hadn't read the directions! Later, when I read the product label, I discovered it had all manner of draconian warnings and instructions that, had I read them beforehand, would have made me more cautious when I first applied the Icy Hot—and saved me from what my adult kids now fondly call "the Great Crotch Fire of 1997."

Sadly, none of us are handed a binder with directions for living when we arrive in the world, and even if we were, spiritually stiff-necked people like us probably wouldn't read them, at least not carefully. Thus, many of us end up careening through the world with our pants on fire, not understanding why the pain keeps getting worse. For me, the Twelve Steps are the directions I wish someone had given me earlier in life. In fact, I often wish my kindergarten teacher, Mrs. Shea, had handed me a children's translation of the Twelve Steps, saying, "Here ya go, kid. You'll thank me later." Alas, she didn't.

Again, the Twelve Steps are simple and profound: make peace with God (Steps One to Three), yourself (Steps Four to Seven), and others (Steps Eight and Nine) and cultivate a lifestyle that supports health and growth in each of those important domains (Steps Ten to Twelve). So far, so good! But in Step Twelve, we're given one last set of directions, which we need to read and follow or we will end up with our pants on fire (again) and risk losing everything we've gained. Those last directions can be summarized in one pithy phrase: "You can't keep it if you don't give it away."

How These Steps Bring About a Spiritual Awakening

But first things first. Let's break this Step down. As I said earlier, the purpose of the Twelve Steps is to facilitate a spiritual awakening of sufficient force that it will transform your personality (the way you habitually act, think, feel, and see the world), swap out your need for an addictive substance or behavior for a relationship with God (which is what you were looking for all along anyway), and profoundly change your way of moving through the world.

Diligently working a program of recovery will empower you to manage the inescapable pain of life—from stepping in a pile of dog mess to IRS audits—without having to resort to your fave addiction(s) to dodge the uncomfortable feelings these experiences arouse. It will profoundly alter the way you experience and relate to God, yourself, and others. We're told this awakening is the result of "working these Steps." But what does a spiritual awakening look like, and how can you be sure you've actually had one?

There are as many different kinds of spiritual awakenings as there are people who have them. Though some people have sudden and dramatic spiritual experiences, we shouldn't expect that to always be the case. I'm sorry, but the '80s band Kool & the Gang probably won't magically appear in your kitchen and start playing their hit song "Celebration" when you finally hit your bottom and turn your will and your life over to the care of God. If they do, let me know. It'd be a first. No, most spiritual awakenings happen gradually for folks as they progress through the Steps. In fact, most spiritual awakenings are so subtle and incremental that others will see a transformation in the way you show up for life before you do.

"You seem more grounded and peaceful." "You're less serious and hard on yourself than in the past." "I feel like you're more present and compassionate than you used to be." "Whatever it is you've found, I want it too." These are just a few of the kind things people said to me as I worked through the Steps in my first year of sobriety. That others saw and commented on my becoming a happier, more spiritually sane person was confirmation that the Steps worked and inspired me to continue on the path of recovery.

All to say, don't fret if you don't have an immediate tornadic spiritual experience deserving of an appendix to the book of Revelation. In my experience, God works more secretly than seismically in our depths.

That being said, here's a sure sign you're undergoing a spiritual overhaul—you will begin to realize and enjoy the fact that you're no longer the center of the universe. You will miraculously begin to acquire and enjoy the virtues of self-forgetfulness and humility.

"Selfishness—self-centeredness! That, we think, is the root of our troubles."[3] Bill Wilson said that, and boy, was he right. The untamed ego is an overinflated, insecure, easily offended, and self-obsessed creature. Not sure? Who is the first person you look for in a group photo taken at your twenty-fifth high school class reunion? *You!* And once you locate yourself in the photo, you start to assess how you stack up against everyone else in the picture, right? *Man, Jim has put on a few pounds, eh? I look like Hugh Jackman next to him.* Then you might think, *Oh, there's Linda. She didn't say a word to me that whole night. She was always such a snob.* That's right, the ego always draws attention to itself. It constantly compares itself to others and lusts for external validation. Seriously, it won't shut up. When it's not lavishing praise on itself, it's tearing itself apart for not measuring up. Is it any wonder we turn to medicating behaviors to quiet it down? We're egomaniacs with inferiority complexes, for goodness' sake!

I once was an easily discouraged person who was prone to bouts of self-pity. When I threw a "pity party," it involved caterers, valet parking, and a tent rental. But as I've worked the program, I'm finally finding freedom from "the bondage of self [ego]."[4] To borrow a phrase from Tim Keller, now I don't think more of myself nor less of myself; instead, *I think of myself less.*[5] I wish I could take credit for this continuing transformation (I still have a long way to go), but I can't. It's simply what happens when we abandon ourselves to God, face the hard and marvelous truths about ourselves, make peace with others, and commit to a spiritual path that compassionately monitors and rightsizes our ego—in other words, when we work the Steps.

Now look, I'm a priest and a therapist. I want you to have a healthy self-esteem and positive self-regard, but every great spiritual master makes the same claim—to find true and lasting joy you have to stop thinking everything is about *you.* You have to get over your "self."

And once you do, your ego becomes your friend. It no longer has anything to prove or disprove. It's content to rest in the inexhaustible love of God. Now you find you no longer overidentify with the younger son in the parable of the prodigal and begin to look and act more like his father, dispensing love, mercy, forgiveness, and grace on others. This is a sure sign you're in the midst of a true awakening of the spirit, and that you're ready for the next piece of Step Twelve—to seek to carry this message to everyone, for the truth is that to keep your recovery, you have to give it away.

I once heard a story about a hip young couple from Manhattan who quit their high-flying jobs, sold their swanky loft in Soho, and bought a farm in Vermont to escape the rat race and open a bed-and-breakfast. (This is a well-rehearsed script for naive urbanites that rarely ends well, but I digress.) One day, the DIY-challenged couple discovered that the water in their well smelled and tasted disgusting. When they asked their crusty neighbor for help, he asked, "When was the last time you drew water from the well?" "Ages ago," they replied. "We're living in a rental while we rehab the house." "That's the problem," the neighbor said, shaking his head at the ignorant city slickers. "If you don't use a well, the water goes bad."

The same rules apply to Twelve-Step spirituality. If you don't regularly draw water from the well of your newfound recovery and share the miracle of what you've found with others, then you'll soon be back where you started. Though it may sound counterintuitive (most gospel ideas do), sharing what you've been given with others is partly motivated by self-interest. The only way to keep what you have is to give it away. As Bill Wilson wrote, "Practical experience shows that nothing will so much insure immunity from drinking [or any other addiction] as intensive work with other alcoholics [addicts]."[6]

Service to others takes many forms. If you're a member of an established Twelve-Step recovery community (Alcoholics Anonymous, Overeaters Anonymous, Gamblers Anonymous, Al-Anon, Sex and Love Addicts Anonymous, and so forth), this service can include driving newcomers to meetings, becoming a sponsor, making coffee, setting up the meeting room, helping people feel welcome, listening and offering words of encouragement to people when they need it, and sharing your recovery story with someone who asks to hear it.

But the practice of serving others extends well beyond meeting rooms. Again, the Steps are a total life program. You must be on the lookout to love and serve others everywhere you go—at home, at the office, or whenever the opportunity arises.

Practice These Principles in All Our Affairs

In the rooms of recovery, we're taught that the Steps will not only help us kick our psychological or physical dependency on alcohol, drugs, porn, or whatever our "fix of choice" is, but also that they encapsulate timeless spiritual principles that we want to practice "in all our affairs." We no longer want our egos or riotous instincts to dictate how we live our lives. Now we're living life on a spiritual rather than a self-centered basis. Our main concern now is character development and living lives that are useful, purposeful, and spent in service to others. Simply put, we want to constellate our lives around the spiritual principles embedded in each of the Steps.

STEP ONE
**We admitted we were powerless over _____
—that our lives had become unmanageable.**

> *"Our admissions of personal powerlessness finally turn out to be firm bedrock upon which happy and purposeful lives may be built." (Twelve Steps and Twelve Traditions)*[7]

In Step One, we learn about the spiritual principle of *honesty*. We can't recover if we don't get real and admit that we're *powerless* over our addictions and self-sabotaging behaviors (i.e., we can't stop repeating them by virtue of sheer willpower), and that our internal and external lives are a bit of a mess—if not "a lot of a mess." Getting honest is a nonnegotiable on the path to recovery. I beg you to reflect deeply on your life and honestly face the truth: to believe you're in control of your life and addictions and have it all together is an illusion.

Remember, the Twelve Steps are a full life makeover. The spiritual principle of honesty should pervade your whole person. For example, living by the spiritual principle of honesty means not keeping secrets and always telling the truth to God, yourself, and others. I consciously practice the First Step every day. For instance, I used to find it all too easy to tell people I was late for lunch because there was an accident on the interstate rather than admit that I left the house late because I was trimming my nose hair and lost track of time. Now when I catch myself about to tell even a small lie, I hear my Inner Observer say, *Ahem*, and I quickly cop to the truth. This is no small thing. If we get in the habit of being secretive (like I was in my active addiction) or comfortable with telling "little lies," we will gradually become okay with telling bigger and bigger ones.

STEP TWO
Came to believe that a Power greater than ourselves could restore us to sanity.

> *"As soon as a man [woman] can say that he [she] does believe, or is willing to believe, we emphatically assure him [her] that he [she] is on his [her] way."* (The Big Book)[8]

In Step Two, we embrace the spiritual principle of *hope*. Living on the basis of hope means you now believe in the possibility that you're not on your own down here. There's an intelligent, personal, loving, and trustworthy power in the universe who cares about you and who wants to do for you what you've never been able to do for yourself—namely, transform you into the highest expression of yourself, albeit slowly. The principle of hope also extends to the possibility that maybe, just maybe, this same God can give you the strength and tools you need to accept life on life's terms without chemically or behaviorally numbing yourself.

STEP THREE
Made a decision to turn our will and our lives over to the care of God as we understood Him.

> *"Faith has to work twenty-four hours a day in and through us, or we perish." (The Big Book)*[9]

In Step Three, we discover the principle of *faith*. Faith is believing that no matter what happens, *God has you*. In a 1996 interview, the renowned scholar of world religions Huston Smith summarized what he had learned from his parents as he was growing up: "We are in good hands."[10] Well, that pretty much sums it up for me. Faith is trusting that God is at the helm, and therefore we don't have to be. Said another way, I may be powerless, but God isn't. If I daily turn my will and my life over to his care, then "all shall be well, all shall be well, and all manner of things shall be well," as the Christian mystic Julian of Norwich wrote.[11] It might sound Pollyannish, but I believe this to my core.

STEP FOUR

**Made a searching and fearless moral
inventory of ourselves.**

"The verdict of the ages is that faith means courage."
(The Big Book)[12]

The principle associated with Step Four is *courage*. You need a steel backbone to voluntarily walk into your shadow to face difficult truths about yourself on a regular basis. But it must be done! I'm daily amazed by my capacity for denial, self-deception, and self-delusion. As Thomas Merton once wrote, "There is no greater disaster in the spiritual life than to be immersed in unreality."[13] As people in recovery who aspire to become higher expressions of ourselves, we have to regularly examine our behaviors, character defects, and motives, or our baser natures will "bust outta their cages" and leave a yard sale of wreckage in their wake.

To be clear, if regularly reviewing your life leaves you feeling ashamed and self-loathing, then something is wrong. Honestly, I expect myself to fail. It's what humans do! Thus, I bring a healthy dose of self-compassion and even humor to my inventories. I also make sure I catalog and applaud my character assets and personal growth when I perform my nightly self-review. I often say, and aspire to live by, the prayer of the Benedictine nun Macrina Wiederkehr, "O God, help me to believe the truth about myself no matter how beautiful it is!"[14]

STEP FIVE

Admitted to God, to ourselves, and to another human being the exact nature of our wrongs.

"Integrity is the state of being fully integrated: Our actions, our thinking, our feelings, our ideals, and our values all match up." (Narcotics Anonymous Living Clean)[15]

Step Five encapsulates the principle of *integrity*. For me, integrity means aligning my insides with my outside. It has to do with being clear about my values and putting them in practice. Embodying integrity means being morally grounded and consistently behaving in an ethical manner. The Buddhists call this "right action." My friend Ari calls it being a *mensch*. Whatever you term it, to have integrity is to be a person of upstanding moral character.

Interestingly, the word *integrity* derives from the Latin word *integritas*, which means "wholeness." Most, if not all, people live fractured, kaleidoscopic lives. All of us don masks and change colors like a chameleon to become whoever it is we think others want us to be so that they'll like and accept us. But if we dissemble for too long, we'll wake up and look in the mirror one day and have no idea who it is that's staring back at us. As Nathaniel Hawthorne wrote in *The Scarlet Letter* (your favorite novel from middle school), "No man, for any considerable period, can wear one face to himself, and another to the multitude, without finally getting bewildered as to which may be the true."[16] No one needs this kind of confusion in their lives.

STEP SIX
**Were entirely ready to have God remove
all these defects of character.**

*"Willingness, honesty, and open mindedness are the essentials
of recovery." (The Big Book)*[17]

Step Six introduces us to the all-important spiritual principle
of *willingness*. Once, while on a trip, I started my rental car
and put it in drive, only to see it violently lunge forward and
screech to a halt. When I pressed the gas a second time, the
car bucked like a bronco and stopped again. Now, I'm not a
"car guy." I couldn't tell you the difference between a glove
compartment and an alternator. But my first thought was that
the transmission was shot. When the nineteen-year-old AAA
guy arrived on the scene, however, he didn't pop the hood
and inspect the engine. No, he got in the driver's seat, looked
around, and then pushed a button on the underside of the
dash. "Your emergency brake was on," he said in a withering
voice. At which point, I handed him twenty bucks and told
him to forget he ever saw me.

Often while working a Twelve-Step program we find ourselves stuck and unable to move forward. When this happens,
we might need to release the brake holding our recovery back
by adopting a greater attitude of willingness to have God
remove our defects of character. "Desperation can get you
started on the road to recovery, but only willingness can keep
you on it," as my friend Jayne likes to say.

We have to be willing to work the Steps (as they're

written, thank you), willing to let go of old character defenses, willing to be humble, willing to ask for help, willing to be vulnerable, to go to meetings, to be of service, to take suggestions and follow directions from our sponsors, to try on new behaviors, to do *anything* to achieve emotional sobriety and get our lives back in order. Let's face it, all of your so-called "best ideas" have gotten you nowhere. But if you let go of your mistaken notions and become willing to have God remove all of your most cherished character defects, then things will change.

STEP SEVEN
Humbly asked Him to remove our shortcomings.

"A great turning point in our lives came when we sought for humility as something we really wanted, rather than as something we must have." (Twelve Steps and Twelve Traditions)[18]

Step Seven encapsulates the principle of *humility*, an indispensable virtue for anyone who wants to recover from their addictions or self-medicating behaviors and live a "happy, joyous, and free" life.[19] It's no coincidence that the words *humor* and *humility* derive from the same word in Latin, *humus*, meaning "earth" or "soil." For me, the shared origin of the two words implies that humble people know how to laugh at themselves.

One of the things that surprises newcomers to the rooms of recovery is how much hilarity and laughter there are in our meetings. Sure, we have our tearful, heartfelt moments, but if you go to a Twelve-Step meeting that's overly earnest and gloomy, run for the hills and find another one. As my friend Curt Thompson once said to me, "The laughter one hears in the rooms of recovery is proof that the pain of addiction doesn't get to have the last word; God does."[20]

It's vital to take your recovery seriously, but not *yourself*. A humble person easily rolls their eyes at their foibles and follies and never misses an opportunity to laugh at their own expense.

As pastor Ted Loder says: "Laughter is a holy thing. It is as sacred as music and silence and solemnity, maybe more sacred. Laughter is like a prayer, like a bridge over which creatures tiptoe to meet each other. Laughter is like mercy; it heals. When you can laugh at yourself, you are free."[21]

STEP EIGHT

Made a list of all persons we had harmed, and became willing to make amends to them all.

> "If we are now about to ask forgiveness for ourselves, why shouldn't we start out by forgiving them, one and all?" (*Twelve Steps and Twelve Traditions*)[22]

The spiritual principle that correlates to Step Eight is *forgiveness*. Several years ago, I was asked to serve as Archbishop Desmond Tutu's chaplain for a few days while he was on a US speaking tour (in the Anglican tradition, *chaplain* is a fancy word for *runner*). My job was to accompany the archbishop to his events and make sure he had everything he needed.

It was a privilege to spend personal time with Archbishop Tutu, the recipient of the Nobel Peace Prize for his role in opposing and ending apartheid in South Africa. Before meeting him, I assumed a man who had witnessed and experienced as much suffering as he had at the hands of others would be solemn, but that's the last thing Tutu was. The man radiated joy! He delighted in telling jokes and cackled at every opportunity! Once, while processing down the aisle of a packed church, he grabbed my hand and made me dance with him to the strains of the rousing opening hymn. Later, when I read his book *No Future without Forgiveness*, I understood the source of the archbishop's gleeful spirit: He had forgiven his perpetrators. He was free.

All of us have experienced hurt at the hands of others. Many of us turned to addictive behaviors to drown unresolved feelings of pain and resentment toward those who wronged us in the past. In recovery, we come to understand that no one is unforgivable or undeserving of forgiveness, including ourselves. We must forgive, or we will be forever trapped in a "labyrinth of suffering"[23] and risk losing our sobriety. Whenever we're hurt, we seek to forgive and move on with our lives.

STEP NINE
Made direct amends to such people wherever possible, except when to do so would injure them or others.

"Love and tolerance of others is our code." (The Big Book)[24]

In Step Nine, we make a commitment to reconcile with those we've hurt. The spiritual principle at work here is *love*.

The teacher Tara Brach tells a marvelous parable about a prickle of porcupines (yup, that's what they're called) facing the harshest winter on record. It was so cold that many animals in the forest froze to death. To stave off the subzero temperatures, the porcupines decided to huddle together to share their body heat. What the porcupines didn't factor into their plan, however, was the pain and annoyance caused by their sharp quills stabbing and pricking each other. Soon, the discomfort of being in such close proximity to each other proved intolerable. Many porcupines abandoned the group and wandered into the night, only to freeze to death alone. Eventually, the remaining porcupines realized they faced a choice. They could stay together and learn to accept their spiky companions, or they could die in the cold. Wisely, they banded together again. To stay warm and survive, they learned to forgive the unavoidable jabs and wounds caused by their companions' quills.[25]

Human beings are prickly creatures. We frequently say and do things that annoy and wound our fellows. There's no way around it. Bill Wilson underscored the need to extend grace, courtesy, patience, and kindness toward those who bother or injure us. As he wrote in *The Big Book*, "Love and tolerance of others is our code." Thankfully, the Steps give us the tools we need to live by the spiritual principle of love. We learn not to take things personally. We shrug off small offenses. And most importantly, we're taught to quickly make amends to those we've hurt so we can enjoy close relationships with others.

STEP TEN

Continued to take personal inventory and when we were wrong promptly admitted it.

> *"As we persist, a brand-new kind of confidence is born, and the sense of relief at finally facing ourselves is indescribable."* (Twelve Steps and Twelve Traditions)[26]

The spiritual principle encapsulated in Step Ten is *perseverance*. No one has taught me more about this virtue than my personal trainer and friend, Juan Carlos. JC, as he likes to be called, is a jocular, thirty-five-year-old guy who looks like he can bench-press a Volvo. Several mornings a week, he drags me into the gym and pushes my body to its limits.

Sin dolor, no hay gloria! (without pain, there is no glory!), he yells at me in Spanish while I swing battle ropes or perform burpees under his watchful gaze. At the end of every session, he smiles and squeezes my puny biceps with his giant hand, saying, "You're getting stronger, Ian. But, of course, you need to come back tomorrow."

Every morning when I wake up, I say my prayers and remind myself that I can't afford to take a day off from my recovery. If I don't remain focused and vigilant about working the Steps and living a healthy, mindful lifestyle, I risk slipping back into old addictive and self-defeating behaviors. Surely, the biblical writer James had addicts like me in mind when he wrote, "Let perseverance finish its work so that you may be mature and complete, not lacking anything" (1:4).

When I do my daily personal inventory in bed at night,

I realize I still have work to do. I'm getting stronger "But, of course, I still need to come back tomorrow" and recommit to working my program of recovery with dogged determination.

STEP ELEVEN

Sought through prayer and meditation to improve our conscious contact with God as we understood Him, praying only for knowledge of His will for us and the power to carry that out.

"So, practicing these Steps, we had a spiritual awakening about which finally there was no question." (Twelve Steps and Twelve Traditions)[27]

The spiritual principle encapsulated in Step Eleven is *spiritual awakeness*—waking up and staying awake. Of course, this idea that all of us suffer from a "spiritual sleep disorder" isn't original to Bill Wilson. As the apostle Paul writes in Romans, "The hour has already come for you to wake up from your slumber, because our salvation is nearer now than when we first believed" (Romans 13:11).

For me, "waking up" means seeing and rejoicing in God's presence in everyone and everything that happens in my life. Unfortunately, spiritual awakeness isn't our default setting. We're on cruise control most of the time. Waking up can be unpleasant and irritating. We are nice and comfortable sleeping in the beds of our routines and small daily concerns and forget that "the world is charged with the grandeur of God," as the poet Gerard Manley Hopkins wrote.[28]

It's only through improving our conscious contact with God through regular prayer and meditation that we can resist repeatedly hitting the snooze button so we can emerge out of our spiritual torpor to see what God is up to in the world and join him in his work.

STEP TWELVE

Having had a spiritual awakening as the result of these Steps, we tried to carry this message to alcoholics [our fellow sufferers], and to practice these principles in all our affairs.

> *"Our real purpose is to fit ourselves to be of maximum service to God and the people about us." (The Big Book)*[29]

When you reach Step Twelve, you realize that the goal of working the Steps was never merely to stop drinking, drugging, control-freaking, shopping, overeating, or whatever it is you do to anesthetize the madness of your inner world. The goal was to have a spiritual awakening that produces a life dedicated to helping others on their own paths to becoming more whole human beings. We now live according to the spiritual principle of *service*.

My seventy-year-old friend Seth has been in recovery for forty-three years. Whether speaking to an old friend or a brand-new acquaintance, he ends every conversation by asking the person, "Is there anything specific I can do to be of service to you or your family?" I've witnessed him pose this question to people numerous times, and it always blows people away.

The reason? Seth is utterly sincere! If a person makes a request, he immediately notes it on his iPhone and does everything he can to quickly follow through on whatever he promised he'd do. Trust me, I've heard incredible anecdotes about the things Seth has done for people.

Spiritually speaking, Seth is a deep well, a man who has done the work. He doesn't offer to serve others to win their approval or because he doesn't know how to set appropriate boundaries. His offers of help are altruistic, not self-interested. When I asked him once what inspired him to start this practice, he quoted the Jesuit priest Michael Graham: "Service is what prayer looks like when it gets up off its knees and walks around in the world."[30] The Twelve Steps intend to bring about in us a spiritual awakening and a life of radical self-donation and serving love.

EPILOGUE

That's what life's all about: little by little, day by day, with excruciating stubbornness, each of us learning how to be less screwed up.
Dean Koontz, *Icebound*

It was a Rockwellian October morning when I first visited A.A. founder Bill Wilson's grave in East Dorset, Vermont. The sky was cerulean blue; the tips of the towering maples were flaring orange and red; and the air was hazy from the smoke wafting from nearby chimneys, sweetening the crisp, cool autumn air.

No other soul was in the hillside cemetery that day, and I was worried I wouldn't be able to find Bill's final resting place. Thankfully, his gravesite stands out, not because it's conspicuously grand, but because it's covered with bouquets of flowers, stuffed animals, and other gifts left by people who, like me, have made the pilgrimage to his last home to say thank you.

If you had been with me that day, the first thing you would have noticed was how modest his headstone is. There's no mention on it that he founded Alcoholics Anonymous or that he conceived the spiritual program called the Twelve Steps, which has saved the lives of countless millions, including my own. All that is etched on it is "Bill Wilson, 1895–1971."

And there are letters of appreciation on Bill's grave as well, weighted down by stones to prevent them from blowing away. These poignant notes come from parents, children, spouses, partners, siblings, and friends of people who have found a second chance at life because of the Twelve Steps and the many programs of recovery. One person wrote these words:

Dear Bill,

For eight years our daughter was lost. Thanks to God and you, now she's found.

Sincerely, a grateful father

What I saw next broke me. Many Twelve-Step recovery groups have a tradition of handing out poker chip–sized brass medallions at the end of meetings to people celebrating months or years of continuous sobriety. It's always a highlight when the chairperson asks if anyone is celebrating a sobriety anniversary, and birthday celebrants come up to receive a hug and their chip as fellow members cheer and applaud their milestones. And there, atop Bill's headstone, were stacks of sobriety chips—marking anniversaries ranging from one month to fifty-five years—left by redeemed souls as a gesture of gratitude. And I wept.

The Twelve Steps saved and restored me to life, and I hope now you realize they can do the same for you. The Twelve Steps are for anyone—not just alcoholics and drug addicts. They're a spiritual program for living that works for everybody.

I have a framed cartoon from *The New Yorker* on my office desk showing a Bedouin family riding on camels in the Sahara Desert. The father is in front, followed by his travel-weary wife, and their three kids on smaller camels taking up the rear. In the cartoon, the father looks over his shoulder and yells at the kids, "Stop asking if we're almost there yet. We're nomads, for crying out loud!"

This whimsical cartoon reminds me that we're all nomads on the spiritual journey. There's no point in asking, "Are we almost there yet?" because we'll never get *there* (wherever "there" is), at least not on this bank of the great divide. Please don't believe the authors of those happy-clappy, self-help books who triumphantly proclaim you can achieve "your best life ever." You're not *there* yet. And whatever you do, don't listen to those sweaty-jowled prosperity preachers who promise that you can attain "the life you've always wanted." Nope, you're not *there* yet.

Your occasional restlessness and disquiet won't be going away anytime soon. You will never completely heal in this life from the pain, losses, and disappointments you suffered in your childhood. There will always be seasons when your marriage and career feel beige and unsatisfying. Oh, and your crazy uncle Carl will *always* show up on Christmas with a gift basket full of near-psychedelic conspiracy theories. It's just how things are.

Sure, there will be halcyon days when the Big Ache and that old "not-at-home" feeling recede into the background, and you will feel momentarily carefree. I've had more of those days than I deserve. But trust me, the Big Ache will always be there.

But don't despair. There's hope for us mortals yet!

For many years, I met regularly with a spiritual director named Brother Gary, an Episcopal monk who lives in a monastery in Cambridge, Massachusetts. Clad in a black cowl and wearing delicate wire-rimmed glasses on his cherubic face, Gary is soft-spoken and composed, and he oozes empathy—everything you imagine a monastic would be. During COVID-19, Brother Gary and I met over Zoom one afternoon for spiritual direction. On that day, I was in a particularly churlish mood. I whined and complained to him about *everything*—from my feral childhood to the pernicious deer in my backyard eating our honeysuckle. As I said, Brother Gary is usually self-possessed and patient, but I can make even the saintliest monk want to poke me in the eye when I'm acting like a dolt.

"Ian," he said sharply, leaning into his computer's camera so that his face overtook my whole screen. "This is *your* life. *These* are the cards. What's the invitation?"

What Brother Gary was attempting to do was get me to wake up and see that an invitation from God is always embedded in our trials, a summons to "get over ourselves," to bravely look our lives straight in the eye and make something better out of them. We're on this earth to learn how to "bear the beams of love," as William Blake wrote,[1] to lean into the Spirit, to avail ourselves of healing, to ease the burdens of others, and not rely on overeating, drinking, drugging, watching porn, compulsively controlling people, or any other repetitive, self-medicating behaviors to escape reality and make life more tolerable—which they *absolutely* never do. To accept this challenge and take responsibility for your own life is "the Work," as therapists and spiritual masters say. In my tribe, we call this pursuit "recovery."

The Twelve Steps have taught me a lot more than how not to drink or use drugs. Abstaining from our addictions and self-destructive behaviors is only the beginning of the Twelve-Step adventure. The Steps are a tool that has taught me how to suit up, show up, and grow up. They've revealed that life only makes sense when we surrender; make peace with our higher power, ourselves, and others; and then cultivate a lifestyle that protects and nurtures these relationships. It's hard, so we take it one day at a time.

Practicing the Twelve Steps has also shown me that happiness and serenity come when I can look at my circumstances and say to myself, *This is how things are. I accept life on life's terms.* To be clear, acceptance is not resignation. Resigned people are a glum lot. They ruefully walk around acting as though life owed them something but failed to keep its end of the bargain.

But here's the paradox—when you finally cease fighting everything and everyone and acknowledge you're not in charge, you discover the courage, serenity, hope, and love for life that your heart longed for all along. As M. Scott Peck famously wrote, "Life is difficult. This is a great truth, one of the greatest truths. It is a great truth because once we truly see this truth, we transcend it. Once we truly know that life is difficult—once we truly understand and accept it—then life is no longer difficult. Because once it is accepted, the fact that life is difficult no longer matters."[2]

I'm talking real freedom here, people.

Now, when the universe refuses to get on board with all of my wonderful plans for my life or when the Big Ache comes calling, I don't reach for a fix in the form of a drink, a drug, or an Oreo, or start people-pleasing or status-seeking, or whatever. Instead, I reach for the Twelve Steps and acceptance. I ask, *What does love require of me right now?* and I steer myself in that direction.

These days, I keep my recovery on speed dial. I call on the Twelve Steps multiple times a day. I wanted a new life, and it has been granted to me. I once was lost and now am found. And for that, I say, "Thanks be to God."

ACKNOWLEDGMENTS

- First and foremost, to my wife, Anne. If not for you, I wouldn't be able to remember why I walked into half the rooms in our house, much less write a book. I love you.
- To my children, Cail, Maddie, and Aidan.
- To Steve Lee, for teaching me how to "trudge the road of happy destiny."
- To my kind, wise, and ever-encouraging literary agent Kathy Helmers.
- To my whip-smart editor Keren Baltzer, my production editor Dirk Buursma, my publisher Webb Younce, and the Zondervan sales and marketing team for their commitment to getting this book into the hands of as many humans as possible.
- To my beloved team and friends—Wendy Nyborg, Lance Villio, and Anthony Skinner.
- To my friends in the "Do It All for the Cookie" club—you know who you are.
- To all the fine souls at Cirque Lodge.
- To my dear brothers and sisters Michael Cusick and Peter Zaremba, Josh Graves, Chris and Laurel Scarlata, Rob Mathes, Steve and Debbie Taylor, Mary Gauthier, Becca Stevens, Scott Owings, Ashley Cleveland, Jayne and Drew Morris, Kathy Lenze, Matt Murphy, Graham Bramblett, Craig Paschal, Forbes Smallwood.
- And, of course, to Percy and Pippa—my canine muses.

ABOUT THE AUTHOR

Ian Morgan Cron is a bestselling author, psychotherapist, Enneagram teacher, trained spiritual director, and Episcopal priest. As someone who works a Twelve-Step program, he's a knowledgeable, compassionate, and humorous guide on the road to recovery. Ian accepts a limited number of private coaching clients to thoughtfully guide them on their personal and professional path. He and his wife, Anne, live in Nashville, Tennessee.

Find out more at ianmorgancron.com.

NOTES

Chapter 1: Desperate for a Fix

1. William Shakespeare, *Hamlet*, act 1, scene 4, line 90.
2. Ethan Nichtern, *The Road Home: A Contemporary Exploration of the Buddhist Path* (New York: North Point, 2015), 4.
3. Anne Porter, *Living Things* (Hanover, NH: Steerforth, 2006), 54.
4. See C. S. Lewis, *The Weight of Glory: And Other Addresses* (1949; repr., San Francisco: HarperOne, 2001), 31.
5. Gerald May, *Addiction and Grace* (San Francisco: HarperOne, 1998), 11.
6. This concept of addictions as idolatry is from Gerald May's wonderful book *Addiction and Grace*, 13.
7. Richard Rohr and Andreas Ebert, *The Enneagram: A Christian Perspective* (New York: Crossroad, 2001), 10.
8. Gabor Maté, "What Is Addiction?," YouTube, January 7, 2014, www.youtube.com/watch?v=T5sOh4gKPIg.
9. Quoted in Conrad W. Baars, *Born Only Once: The Miracle of Affirmation*, 3rd ed. (Eugene, OR: Wipf & Stock, 2016), 18.
10. Bill W., *Alcoholics Anonymous: The Story of How Many Thousands of Men and Women Have Recovered from Alcoholism*, 4th ed. (New York: Alcoholics Anonymous World Services, 2001), 27.
11. Bill W., *Alcoholics Anonymous*, 25.

Chapter 2: Drinking from the Wrong Well

1. Anne Lamott, *Imperfect Birds: A Novel* (New York: Penguin, 2010), 192.
2. "Appendix D: Important Facts about Alcohol and Drugs," in *Facing Addiction in America: The Surgeon General's Report on Alcohol, Drugs, and Health*, U.S. Department of Health and Human Services, November 2016, www.ncbi.nlm.nih.gov /books/NBK424847.
3. Anne Lamott, *Bird by Bird: Some Instructions on Writing and Life* (New York: Anchor, 1994), 93.
4. Cited in Tracy Hampton, "Study Holds Warning on Pandemic Drinking," *Harvard Gazette*, January 4, 2022, https://news.harvard.edu/gazette/story/2022/01/covid -related-drinking-linked-to-rise-in-liver-disease.
5. Brené Brown, "The Power of Vulnerability," TED, June 2010 (15:29–33), www.ted.com/talks/brene_brown_the_power _of_vulnerability.
6. Sister Mary Colombiere, "Spiritual Detachment," Carmelite Sisters of the Most Sacred Heart of Los Angeles, September 16, 2012, https://carmelitesistersocd.com/2012 /spiritual-detachment.
7. The story of the skylark is paraphrased from an article in a New Zealand newspaper titled "Wings for Worms," *The Evening Star*, September 8, 1917, https://paperspast.natlib .govt.nz/newspapers/ESD19170908.2.9.
8. Gabor Maté, *In the Realm of Hungry Ghosts: Close Encounters with Addiction* (Berkeley, CA: North Atlantic, 2008), 1.
9. Adapted from C. S. Lewis, *The Great Divorce* (1946; repr., New York: HarperOne, 2001), 106–15.
10. W. H. Auden, *The Age of Anxiety: A Baroque Eclogue*, ed. Alan Jacobs (Princeton: Princeton University Press, 2011), 105.
11. Bill W., *Alcoholics Anonymous: The Story of How Many Thousands of Men and Women Have Recovered from Alcoholism*,

4th ed. (New York: Alcoholics Anonymous World Services, 2001), 206.

Chapter 3: Without a Paddle

1. "Monty Python and the Holy Grail," directed by Terry Gilliam and Terry Jones (Burbank, CA: Columbia Pictures, 1975), accessed July 29, 2024, https://sfy.ru/?script=mp_holygrail.
2. Dylan Thomas, "Do Not Go Gentle into That Good Night," in *The Poems of Dylan Thompson* (New York: New Directions, 2017).
3. J. R. R. Tolkien coined the word *euchatastrophe* in a 1944 essay, "On Faerie-stories," in *Tolkien on Fairy-stories*, rev. ed., ed. Verlyn Flieger and Douglas A. Anderson (London: HarperCollins, 2014), 75.
4. Ernest Kurtz and Katherine Ketcham, *The Spirituality of Imperfection: Storytelling and the Search for Meaning* (New York: Bantam, 1992), 29, emphasis added.
5. A. W. Tozer, *I Talk Back to the Devil: The Fighting Fervor of the Victorious Christian*, The Tozer Pulpit 4 (1972; repr., Chicago: Moody, 2018), 88.

Chapter 4: Helplessly Hoping

1. Bill W., *Alcoholics Anonymous: The Story of How Many Thousands of Men and Women Have Recovered from Alcoholism*, 4th ed. (New York: Alcoholics Anonymous World Services, 2001), 46.
2. Bill W., *Alcoholics Anonymous*, 46.
3. Paul Greene, "The Set Aside Prayer," Manhattan Center for Cognitive Behavioral Therapy, accessed July 29, 2024, https://manhattancbt.com/set-aside-prayer.
4. Gyles Brandreth, "An Easter Conversation: Going to Heaven with Desmond Tutu," GylesBrandeth.net, March 30, 2018, www.gylesbrandreth.net/blog/2018/3/30/an-easter -conversation-going-to-heaven-with-desmond-tutu#.

5. See Christine Comaford, "Got Inner Peace? 5 Ways to Get It *NOW*," *Forbes*, November 7, 2013, www.forbes.com/sites /christinecomaford/2012/04/04/got-inner-peace-5-ways-to -get-it-now.

6. Michael A. Singer, *The Untethered Soul: The Journey beyond Yourself* (Oakland, CA: New Harbinger, 2007), 16–19.

Chapter 5: Somebody Take the Wheel

1. Bill W., *Alcoholics Anonymous: The Story of How Many Thousands of Men and Women Have Recovered from Alcoholism*, 4th ed. (New York: Alcoholics Anonymous World Services, 2001), 63.

2. Quoted in Judson B. Trapnell, *Bede Griffiths: A Life in Dialogue* (Albany, NY: SUNY Press, 2001), 45.

3. Saint Augustine, *Confessions* 3.6.11 (translation of the Latin *interior intimo meo at superior summon meo*: "You are more inward to me than my most inward part and higher than my highest"); quoted in William Placher, ed., *Essentials of Christian Theology* (Louisville: Westminster John Knox, 2003), 113.

4. Bill W., *Alcoholics Anonymous*, 55.

5. Bill W., *Twelve Steps and Twelve Traditions* (1953; repr., New York: Alcoholics Anonymous World Services, 2001), 106–7.

Chapter 6: Hug the Cactus

1. Thomas Merton, "Hagia Sophia: Dawn," in *In the Dark before Dawn*, ed. Lynn R. Szabo (New York: New Directions, 2005), 65.

2. Bill W., *Alcoholics Anonymous: The Story of How Many Thousands of Men and Women Have Recovered from Alcoholism*, 4th ed. (New York: Alcoholics Anonymous World Services, 2001), 66.

3. "Robert Downey Jr. Asks Forgiveness for Mel Gibson," YouTube, October 18 2011, www.youtube.com /watch?v=_AAJuynxnTQ.

4. Bill W., *Alcoholics Anonymous*, 64.

5. *Pocket Oxford Dictionary of Current English* (Oxford: Oxford University Press, 1996), s.v. "Resentment."

6. C. G. Jung, *Alchemical Studies*, vol. 13 in *Collected Works of C. G. Jung* (Princeton, NJ: Princeton University Press, 1953), 266.

7. Elizabeth Gilbert, *Eat, Pray, Love* (New York: Penguin, 2006), 186.

8. Bill W., *Alcoholics Anonymous*, 65.

9. Bill W., *Alcoholics Anonymous*, 67.

10. Bill W., *Alcoholics Anonymous*, 66.

11. Bill W., *Alcoholics Anonymous*, 66–67.

12. Bill W., *Alcoholics Anonymous*, 58.

13. Bill W., *Alcoholics Anonymous*, 64.

14. Bill W., *Alcoholics Anonymous*, 68.

15. Bill W., *Alcoholics Anonymous*, 69.

16. Frederick Buechner, *Telling Secrets* (San Francisco: HarperOne, 1991), 33.

Chapter 7: Fess Up

1. See n.a., *Experience, Strength, and Hope: Stories from the First Three Editions of* Alcoholics Anonymous (New York: Alcoholics Anonymous World Services, 2003).

2. Bessel van der Kolk, *The Body Keeps the Score: Brain, Mind, and Body in the Healing of Trauma* (New York: Viking, 2014), 234.

3. Keith Miller, *A Hunger for Healing: The Twelve Steps as a Classic Model for Christian Spiritual Growth* (San Francisco: HarperSanFrancisco, 1991), 87.

4. George Appleton, "A Gathering Prayer," in *One Man's Prayers* (London: SPCK, 1967), 13, my paraphrase.

5. Bill W., *Alcoholics Anonymous: The Story of How Many Thousands of Men and Women Have Recovered from Alcoholism*, 4th ed. (New York: Alcoholics Anonymous World Services, 2001), 75.

6. Johann Hari, *Chasing the Scream: The First and Last Days of the War on Drugs* (New York: Bloomsbury, 2015); this quote comes from Johann Hari, "The Opposite of Addiction Isn't Sobriety – It's Connection," *Guardian*, April 12, 2016, www.theguardian.com/books/2016/apr/12/johann-hari-chasing-the-scream-war-on-drugs.

7. Tara Brach, *Radical Acceptance: Embracing Your Life with the Heart of a Buddha* (New York: Bantam, 2003), 5.

8. Bill W., *Alcoholics Anonymous*, 75.

9. Paul Tillich, *The Shaking of the Foundations* (New York: Scribner, 1955), 161–62.

Chapter 8: Okay, I'm Willing Already

1. The story is told in Bill P., Todd W., and Sara S., *Drop the Rock: Removing Character Defects, Steps 6 and 7*, 2nd ed. (Center City, MN: Hazelden, 2005), xi–xii.

2. Bill W., *Twelve Steps and Twelve Traditions* (1953; repr., New York: Alcoholics Anonymous World Services, 2001), 63.

3. Bill W., *Twelve Steps and Twelve Traditions*, 76.

4. Bill W., *Alcoholics Anonymous: The Story of How Many Thousands of Men and Women Have Recovered from Alcoholism*, 4th ed. (New York: Alcoholics Anonymous World Services, 2001), 84.

5. Pierre Teilhard de Chardin, "Patient Trust," quoted in Michael J. Harter, ed., *Hearts on Fire: Praying with Jesuits* (Chicago: Loyola, 2004), 102.

6. Thomas Merton, *New Seeds of Contemplation* (New York: New Directions, 1961), 57.

7. Bill W., *Alcoholics Anonymous*, 76.

8. See, for example, Karen A. Baikie and Kay Wilhelm, "Emotional and Physical Health Benefits of Expressive Writing," *Advances in Psychiatric Treatment* 11, no. 5 (September 2005): 338–46, www.cambridge.org/core/journals/advances-in-psychiatric-treatment/article/emotional-and

-physical-health-benefits-of-expressive-writing/ED2976A61F5
DE56B46F07A1CE9EA9F9F.

9. Bill W., *Alcoholics Anonymous*, 60.

Chapter 9: Mea Culpa

1. Quoted words in this paragraph and in the previous paragraph are taken from Dr. Seuss, *Bartholomew and the Oobleck* (New York: Random House, 1949), 49–50.

2. Bill W., *Alcoholics Anonymous: The Story of How Many Thousands of Men and Women Have Recovered from Alcoholism*, 4th ed. (New York: Alcoholics Anonymous World Services, 2001), 76.

3. Zadie Smith, "Introduction: Somebody in There After All," in *Recitatif: A Story*, Toni Morrison (New York: Borzoi, 1983), xxv.

4. Alice Munro, *The Progress of Love* (New York: Vintage, 1985), 30.

5. Bill W., *Alcoholics Anonymous*, 83–84.

Chapter 10: Look Out!

1. See "Two Pilots Allegedly Fall Asleep on Flight from NYC to Rome as Plane Traveled 38K Feet above Ground," ABC 7 Eyewitness News, June 1, 2022, https://abc7chicago.com /pilots-fall-asleep-pilot-during-flight-ita-airways-sleeping /11915028.

2. Cited in "'More Than Half' of Pilots Have Slept While Flying," BBC News, September 27, 2013, www.bbc.com /news/uk-24296544.

3. "Two Pilots Allegedly Fall Asleep."

4. Bill W., "The Next Frontier: Emotional Sobriety," AA Grapevine, January 1958, https://aainthedesert.org/wp -content/uploads/2019/01/EMOTIONAL-SOBRIETY.pdf.

5. Rumi, "A Mouse and a Frog," in *The Essential Rumi*, trans. Coleman Barks (San Francisco: HarperSanFrancisco, 1995), 80, italics in original.

6. Bill W., *Twelve Steps and Twelve Traditions* (1953; repr., New York: Alcoholics Anonymous World Services, 2001), 90, italics in original.

7. Gregory Knox Jones, *Play the Ball Where the Monkey Drops It: Why We Suffer and How We Can Hope* (San Francisco: HarperSanFrancisco, 2001), 3–4.

8. Bill W., *Twelve Steps and Twelve Traditions*, 88.

Chapter 11: So Help Me God

1. Ronald Rolheiser, *The Holy Longing: The Search for a Christian Spirituality*, rev. ed. (New York: Image, 2009), 74.

2. See Bill W., *Alcoholics Anonymous: The Story of How Many Thousands of Men and Women Have Recovered from Alcoholism*, 4th ed. (New York: Alcoholics Anonymous World Services, 2001), 63, 67, 85, 87–88.

3. See Flannery O'Connor, "Revelation," published in *The Sewanee Review* (Spring 1964).

4. *The Book of Common Prayer* (New York: Seabury, 1977), 136–40.

5. *Book of Common Prayer*, 137.

6. *Book of Common Prayer*, 137.

7. Bill W. "What Is Acceptance?," AA Grapevine, March 1962, https://gugogs.org/2020/04/26/example-post-2.

8. Bill W., *Alcoholics Anonymous*, xxviii.

9. Quoted in Richard Rohr, *Falling Upward: A Spirituality for the Two Halves of Life* (Hoboken, NJ: Wiley, 2011), 66.

10. Julian of Norwich, "The Fourteenth Revelation," chapter 53, in *Revelations of Divine Love* (London: Methuen, 1901), 127–30.

11. Thomas Keating, *Divine Therapy and Addiction: Centering Prayer and the Twelve Steps* (Woodstock, NY: Lantern, 2011).

12. Thomas Merton, *Conjectures of a Guilty Bystander* (New York: Image, 1965), 72.

13. This section on centering prayer is adapted from Rich Lewis, "What Is Centering Prayer? My Discovery of

Centering Prayer," Christian Meditation Center, March 28, 2023, www.christianmeditationcenter.org/what-is-centering-prayer.

14. Father Thomas Keating is cited by Rich Lewis, "My Discovery of Centering Prayer," Christian Meditation Center, March 28, 2023, 1st section.

15. Bill W., *Twelve Steps and Twelve Traditions* (1953; repr., New York: Alcoholics Anonymous World Services, 2001), 96.

Chapter 12: It Works If You Work It

1. David Kuehls, *Four Months to a Four-Hour Marathon* (New York: Perigee, 2006).

2. Phyllis Diller, "New Again: Janeane Garofalo," Interview newsletter, July 29, 2015, www.interviewmagazine.com/culture/new-again-janeane-garofalo.

3. Bill W., *Alcoholics Anonymous: The Story of How Many Thousands of Men and Women Have Recovered from Alcoholism,* 4th ed. (New York: Alcoholics Anonymous World Services, 2001), 62.

4. Bill W., *Alcoholics Anonymous,* 63.

5. See Tim Keller, *The Reason for God: Belief in an Age of Skepticism* (New York: Dutton, 2008), 187.

6. Bill W., *Alcoholics Anonymous,* 89.

7. Bill W., *Twelve Steps and Twelve Traditions* (1953; repr., New York: Alcoholics Anonymous World Services, 2001), 21.

8. Bill W., *Alcoholics Anonymous,* 47.

9. Bill W., *Alcoholics Anonymous,* 16.

10. Quoted in "Remembering Huston Smith, Noted 'World Religions' Scholar," NPR Fresh Air, January 4, 2017, originally aired in 1996, www.npr.org/2017/01/04/508195918/remembering-huston-smith-noted-worlds-religions-scholar.

11. Julian of Norwich, "The Thirteenth Revelation," chapter 27, in *Revelations of Divine Love* (London: Methuen, 1901), 56.

12. Bill W., *Alcoholics Anonymous*, 68.
13. Thomas Merton, *Thoughts in Solitude* (1958; repr., New York: Farrar, Straus and Giroux, 1999), 3.
14. Macrina Wiederkehr O.S.B., *Seasons of Your Heart: Prayers and Reflections* (New York: HarperCollins, 1991), 71.
15. Narcotics Anonymous, *Living Clean: The Journey Continues* (Van Nuys, CA: Narcotics Anonymous World Services, 2012), 37.
16. Nathaniel Hawthorne, *The Scarlet Letter* (Mineola, NY: Dover, 2009), 147.
17. Bill W., *Alcoholics Anonymous*, 568.
18. Bill W., *Twelve Steps and Twelve Traditions*, 75.
19. Bill W., *Alcoholics Anonymous*, 133.
20. Curt Thompson, personal conversation, April 18, 2022.
21. Ted Loder, *Tracks in the Straw: Tales Spun from the Manger* (Minneapolis: Augsburg, 2005), 73.
22. Bill W., *Twelve Steps and Twelve Traditions*, 78.
23. See John Green, *Looking for Alaska* (New York: Penguin, 2015), 103.
24. Bill W., *Alcoholics Anonymous*, 84.
25. See Tara Brach, "Part I: Awakening through Anger – The U-Turn to Freedom," TaraBrach.com, November 11, 2015, www.tarabrach.com/awakening-through-anger-3; see also "5 Lessons to Learn from Porcupines," Amazing Women Rock, accessed July 29, 2024, https://amazingwomenrock .com/the-parable-of-the-prickly-porcupines.
26. Bill W., *Twelve Steps and Twelve Traditions*, 50.
27. Bill W., *Twelve Steps and Twelve Traditions*, 109.
28. Gerard Manley Hopkins, "God's Grandeur," in *Poems and Prose of Gerard Manley Hopkins*, ed. W. H. Gardner (Harmondsworth, UK: Penguin, 1953), 27.
29. Bill W., *Alcoholics Anonymous*, 77.
30. Quoted in "Service Quotes," Xavier University: Jesuit Resource, accessed July 29, 2024, www.xavier.edu/jesuitresource/online -resources/quote-archive1/service-quotes#.

Epilogue

1. William Blake, "The Little Black Boy," Poetry Foundation, accessed July 29, 2024, www.poetryfoundation.org/poems /43671/the-little-black-boy.
2. M. Scott Peck, *The Road Less Traveled: A New Psychology of Love, Traditional Values, and Spiritual Growth* (1978; repr., New York: Touchstone, 2003), 15.

Companion Workbook
Also Available

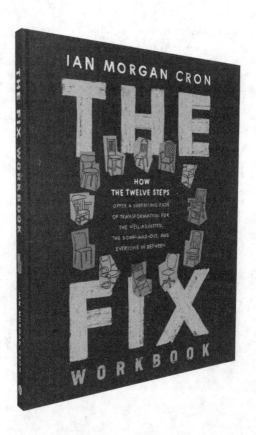

Use alongside the book for
greater understanding.